MW00345875

A JOHNS HOPKINS PRESS HEALTH BOOK

THE **GLAUCOMA GUIDEBOOK**

Expert Advice on
Maintaining Healthy Vision

CONSTANCE OKEKE, MD, MSCE

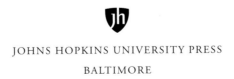

JOHNS HOPKINS UNIVERSITY PRESS

BALTIMORE

Note to the Reader: This book is not meant to substitute for medical care, and treatment should not be based solely on its contents. Instead, treatment must be developed in a dialogue between the individual and their physician. The book has been written to help with that dialogue.

Drug Dosage: The author and publisher have made reasonable efforts to determine that the selection of drugs discussed in this text conform to the practices of the general medical community. The medications described do not necessarily have specific approval by the US Food and Drug Administration for use in the diseases for which they are recommended. In view of ongoing research, changes in governmental regulation, and the constant flow of information relating to drug therapy and drug reactions, the reader is urged to check the package insert of each drug for any change in indications and dosage and for warnings and precautions. This is particularly important when the recommended agent is a new and/or infrequently used drug.

© 2023 Constance Okeke
All rights reserved. Published 2023
Printed in Canada on acid-free paper
2 4 6 8 9 7 5 3 1

Johns Hopkins University Press
2715 North Charles Street
Baltimore, Maryland 21218
www.press.jhu.edu

Library of Congress Cataloging-in-Publication Data

Names: Okeke, Constance, author.
Title: The glaucoma guidebook : expert advice on maintaining healthy vision / Constance Okeke, MD, MSCE
Description: Baltimore : Johns Hopkins University Press, [2023] | Series: A Johns Hopkins Press health book | Includes bibliographical references and index. | Summary: "Dr. Okeke provides a concise guide for readers about glaucoma—an eye disorder that leads to optic nerve damage, vision loss, and blindness. She explains key terms used by doctors to talk about testing and treatment options and provides guidance for readers on how they can take care of their vision as well as their overall health"— Provided by publisher.
Identifiers: LCCN 2022017746 | ISBN 9781421445816 (hardcover) | ISBN 9781421445823 (paperback) | ISBN 9781421445830 (ebook)
Subjects: LCSH: Glaucoma—Popular works. | Glaucoma—Treatment—Popular works.
Classification: LCC RE871 .O34 2023 | DDC 617.7/41--dc23/eng/20220601
LC record available at https://lccn.loc.gov/2022017746

A catalog record for this book is available from the British Library.

Special discounts are available for bulk purchases of this book.
For more information, please contact Special Sales at specialsales@jh.edu.

DISCLAIMER

The mission of the author is to protect the sight and independence of people with glaucoma through education. To this end, the author provides information on glaucoma and glaucoma-related issues. The author works to ensure that the information contained in this book is current, accurate, and useful. Information contained in the book is based on professional advice and expert opinion. This information, however, should not be considered medical guidance or professional advice. The author, her representatives, and any other parties involved in the preparation or publication of this book are not responsible for errors or omissions in the information provided or any actions resulting from the use of such information. Readers are encouraged to confirm the information contained within this book with other reliable sources and to direct any questions concerning their personal health to a licensed eye doctor or other appropriate health care professional.

COPYRIGHT AND REPRINTS

The individual pages provided in this book are copyrighted by Constance Okeke. This information is for personal use only. Permission to otherwise reprint, copy, electronically reproduce, or utilize any document within this book, in part or in whole, is expressly prohibited unless prior written consent is obtained from Constance Okeke.

To request written permission, please email iglaucomapatient@gmail.com.

The compilation of information and materials in this book, including design, graphics, and information, is copyrighted by Constance Okeke. The unauthorized alteration of the content of this book is expressly prohibited. The author and her representatives shall not be responsible for any claims, actions, or damages which may arise as a result of the unauthorized alteration of this book.

FEEDBACK

The author is proud to be a resource on glaucoma and glaucoma-related issues. Let us know what you think about the book. We appreciate your comments and ideas. To send us comments about this book or to request information about our other products, please contact iglaucomapatient@gmail.com.

PROCEEDS BENEFITS

Congratulations!

You are part of the fight against glaucoma blindness.

By purchasing this book, you have just financially contributed to increasing glaucoma awareness, increasing support for glaucoma research, and increasing opportunities for glaucoma surgical care for those in financial need.

The author is donating some of the proceeds of this book's royalties to support the work of the Glaucoma Research Foundation and the American Glaucoma Society's AGS Cares Program. Read more about these organizations and their efforts in the "Philanthropy" section.

Sharing means caring. Spread the word about this book and save sight!

To my husband, Richard,
and my children, Izu, Ify, and Obi,
who support me with love and patience in every effort I make

Contents

Foreword

In this book, Dr. Constance Okeke concludes with the words, "Knowledge is power." I'd like to begin with those same words. With knowledge, fear is eliminated. Dr. Okeke's 12 expert tips help us to understand and take control of our health and glaucoma.

As someone involved with glaucoma for almost 50 years, I've been fortunate to know many of the leading glaucoma specialists around the world and to read many books and articles that help glaucoma patients manage their disease. Dr. Okeke's approach is unique. She keeps her book focused on two themes: understanding and responsibility. *The Glaucoma Guidebook* is an easy book to read and is reassuring through its simple and direct language.

It was at an annual American Glaucoma Society meeting in San Diego where Dr. Okeke and I first met. She was an invited speaker and gave a dynamic and well-received presentation that I still remember. Following the session, I made my way quickly to the front of the room to meet this new speaker with the important message about encouraging glaucoma patients to speak to their family members regarding their increased risk of glaucoma. We had a wonderful conversation and have become friends and colleagues in our mutual efforts to help glaucoma patients preserve their vision through education and research. Dr. Okeke is also an innovator and educator, utilizing the latest technology for the best outcomes for her patients and sharing her experience with other glaucoma specialists through her blogs and training courses.

Robert Shaffer, MD, one of the early glaucoma specialists and a founder of the Glaucoma Research Foundation, taught his glaucoma fellows that it was important to treat the whole patient and not just their glaucoma. As president and CEO of the Glaucoma Research Foundation, I encourage readers to enjoy and learn from Dr. Okeke's guidebook and to take control of their health and glaucoma. Working with their doctors, glaucoma patients can preserve a lifetime of healthy vision.

Knowledge truly is power.

THOMAS M. BRUNNER, BSEE, MBA
President and CEO
Glaucoma Research Foundation

Preface

As we talk about understanding glaucoma, there will be some discussion and use of medical terms. You are in the right place. These medical descriptions are written to help you understand a complex eye disease in simple terms, with pictures to guide that understanding. Again, you are in the right place. By the end of the book, your knowledge and understanding of glaucoma will blossom, and you will gain confidence as you talk to your doctors, family, and friends about glaucoma with your newfound knowledge. Happy reading!

Contributing Editors

Eydie Miller-Ellis, MD
Director of Glaucoma
Professor of Ophthalmology
Scheie Eye Institute
University of Pennsylvania

Samantha Dewundara, MD
Glaucoma Specialist
Virginia Eye Consultants
Assistant Professor of Ophthalmology
Eastern Virginia Medical School

THE GLAUCOMA GUIDEBOOK

Introduction

Dear Reader,

   As a glaucoma specialist, I have words of advice that I'd like to give to every glaucoma patient—words of advice that I've gathered over the years and feel that each patient should know to better take control of their disease.

   Glaucoma is an eye condition that, if left untreated, may lead to blindness. That blindness is irreversible. We know that 50% of the people who have glaucoma are not aware that they actually have the disease, and we know that people who are aware that they have the disease still struggle with trying to live with glaucoma and take care of it.

   Imagine that you lost your vision today. What would you miss most? I want you to take a moment to write it down. Would it be that you would miss looking at the faces of your family members and the memories that you recall having with them? Would it be clear sights that you've seen, particularly if you've traveled around the world and viewed certain beautiful images? Or maybe it would be your independence, being able to take care of yourself, and walking without fear of stumbling or falling. These are things that could actually be lost if your glaucoma is left untreated.

If you have been recently diagnosed with glaucoma, or if you are struggling to manage your glaucoma, this is the book for you. In these pages, you will find some important tips from me—a glaucoma specialist and educator for more than two decades—to you, the glaucoma patient. These tips will help you cope with your diagnosis and treatment and equip you with knowledge to take charge of this serious but treatable eye condition.

All the best,

Constance Okeke, MD, MSCE

1

Understanding Glaucoma

Before we begin to discuss what glaucoma is, I would first like to share with you what the disease looks like. In pictures that try to convey what someone with glaucoma sees, you may be shown an image of normal vision, where the person can visualize everything in the environment (fig. 1.1). Then you'll see a picture of abnormal vision (fig. 1.2), which demonstrates that with glaucoma, there is generally a significant amount of vision lost. This image represents what the world may look like if you have glaucoma, but it is not the same for everyone with the disease.

Glaucoma comes in many different stages, and in its earliest form, people still see and function well. In fact, I've had glaucoma patients who have looked at pictures on my clinic wall, similar to the abnormal one here, and then said, "Oh, I must not have glaucoma, because my vision doesn't look like that." Those patients did have glaucoma, but at a different stage than that of the picture. Unfortunately, this type of thinking is common and can lead to misunderstandings. I'm here to tell you that glaucoma can be very sneaky, subtle, and misleading. In the next section, I will share with you what I believe is a more realistic description of what glaucoma can look like.

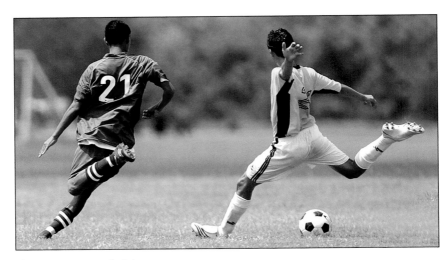

Figure 1.1. Normal vision.

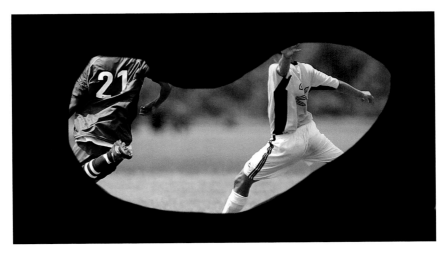

Figure 1.2. The same image viewed by a person with glaucoma.

What Does Glaucoma Look Like? Part 1

A person can have advanced glaucoma and still have 20/20 vision, but their peripheral, or side vision, can be severely affected. This concept of what glaucoma looks like may seem confusing. Let me give you an idea of what glaucoma looks like through two viewpoints.

Viewpoint 1: The Brain Tries to Fuse Both Eye Images

The brain wants you to see your best. It will take the image from each eye individually and then fuse the two together to create the fullest picture. By doing this, it can be easy for you to miss a growing visual deficit in one eye, because the other eye helps pick up the slack. Glaucoma can affect each eye differently. A person can have glaucoma in one eye but not at all in the other eye. On the flip side, a person can have glaucoma in both eyes, but the disease can be worse in one eye compared with the other. Doing the "Cover Your Eyes So You Can See" test can be a great way to pick up on this. See Tip 2 (in chapter 2) for more details.

By looking at the pictures on the next three pages, you can get a better sense of what I mean. These pictures show the viewpoint of a person driving, looking through the front windshield.

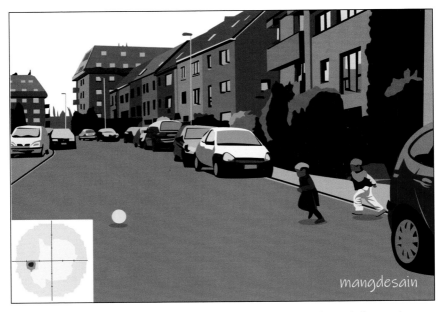

Figure 1.3. A driver's viewpoint with a normal visual field (*lower left corner*), indicating no vision loss.

In the first picture (fig. 1.3), the driver has early-stage glaucoma, with a healthy, full field of vision. The lower left-hand corner contains a diagram for a visual field that is normal. (A visual field is a type of instrument used to measure visual function.) In this setting, the driver can easily see the ball and the two children running after it. Normally, this visual image would allow the driver to see the danger ahead and stop immediately to avoid hitting the children.

I want you to take another look at the picture, noticing a few things in particular:

- The yellow ball in the middle of the street.

- Two kids running after the ball.

- A red car (partial view) in front of kids.

- Tall buildings on both sides of the street.

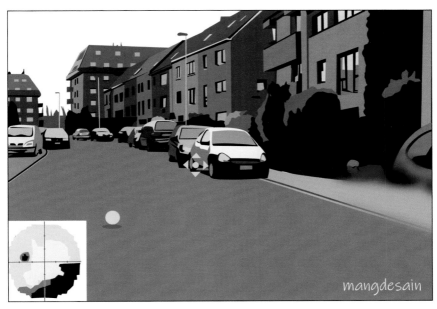

Figure 1.4. A driver's viewpoint with a visual field (*lower left corner*) indicating moderate vision loss due to glaucoma.

In the second picture (fig. 1.4), the viewpoint is the same. Now, however, the driver has moderate-stage glaucoma, with a visual field deficit that affects the field of vision. Can you see where the difference is between the first and second images?

Look again for the yellow ball, the two kids running after it, and the red car near the kids. Notice how the images of the children are gone, except for the top of the head of the boy. Also notice the blurred image of the red car. Glaucoma does not always cause absolute defects that look like stark black blind spots. Some defects are often relative and subtle, like a graying out of the area. *With both eyes open, the brain allows the images to fuse to make up for where there is loss, so the overall image still looks okay.*

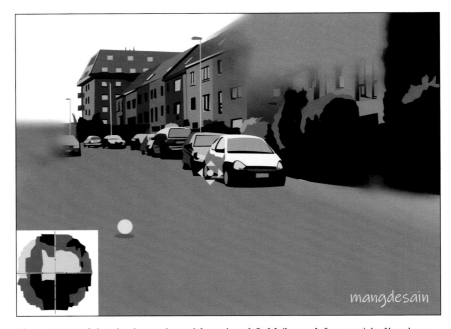

Figure 1.5. A driver's viewpoint with a visual field (*lower left corner*) indicating advanced vision loss due to glaucoma.

In the third picture (fig. 1.5), the driver is now at an advanced stage of glaucoma, although still seeing a clear central image, possibly even with 20/20 vision. The peripheral field, however, is very blurred. Notice, yet again, how the blur is not an absolutely black blind spot. The images are grayed out. Remember the red car? Completely gone now. Remember the buildings on both sides of the street? Now the left-side buildings are gone.

At end-stage glaucoma, your central vision can also be damaged. This is what treatment aims to prevent. We will get to the second viewpoint of what glaucoma looks like after we explain what glaucoma is.

What Is Glaucoma?

Glaucoma is an eye disease that causes damage to a structure in the eye, called the *optic nerve* (fig. 1.6).

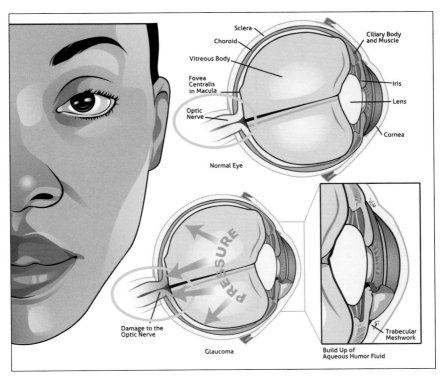

Figure 1.6. Eye anatomy.

This optic nerve is an essential part of the visual pathway. You can think of the optic nerve as a lamp's cable cord and the lamp as the eye. Without the cord, the lamp won't work. If enough damage is done to the optic nerve, it will lead to vision loss. Ultimately, these changes are permanent and can lead to complete blindness if not treated.

Normal Optic Nerve

To understand glaucoma, it is important to know what a normal optic nerve (fig. 1.7) looks like and how it normally works.

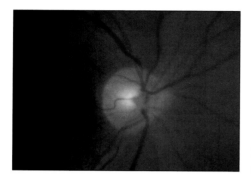

Figure 1.7. A doctor's view of a normal-appearing optic nerve.

When an eye doctor looks into the back of the eye to evaluate it for glaucoma, he or she will look at the optic nerve. The optic nerve typically looks round, like a donut (fig. 1.8). The *disc rim* of the "donut" should be thick. This is an indication that the nerve is healthy, with a robust amount of optic nerve tissue. The central area has a "hole" that we call the *cup*, and this area should be fairly small in size for a normal optic nerve.

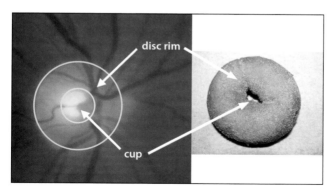

Figure 1.8. *Left*: A normal nerve. *Right*: A donut.

When we are born, the optic nerve is created with a finite amount of nerve cells that make up the disc rim. An average person has about 1.2 to 1.5 million cells. As we age, a small amount of those optic nerve cells will slowly die off. This is normal and expected, because we are typically born with many more nerve cells than we need to last us for a lifetime of good vision.

What happens in glaucoma, however, is that there is a faster rate of loss of those optic nerve cells. If this is left untreated, the loss will begin to cause a permanent decrease of vision, which can significantly impact one's quality of life and ability to function.

Structural Damage in Glaucoma

When nerve cells are lost, the rim of the optic nerve begins to look thin, and the central cup begins to look larger. We call these findings *cupping* of the optic nerve (fig. 1.9). We use a term called *cup-to-disc ratio* when we describe optic nerve cupping. The closer the number is to 0.1, the healthier the nerve; the closer the number is to 1.0, the more diseased the nerve. Findings of increased cupping are of concern because it means there is damage to the nerve tissue. This is disturbing news because nerve tissue loss is permanent. Optic nerve tissue does not grow back and we do not have methods to replenish it.

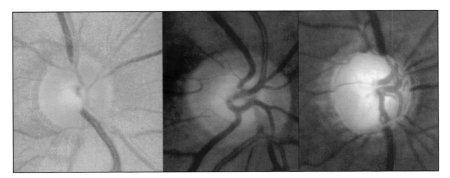

Figure 1.9. Progressive (*left to right*) optic nerve damage.

Functional Damage in Glaucoma

So, what does it mean if you have cupping of the optic nerve? Do you still have normal vision? If you have cupping, there is loss of nerve tissue. Yet you can continue to have normal vision in the early stages of glaucoma. This is why we need to screen further for glaucoma and perform a *visual field test* (fig. 1.10). This test is essentially a map of your visual function. It tells the doctor what you can and cannot see. It can often help determine if glaucoma is present, the stage of the disease, and how aggressive we need to be with treatment. This is a test that should be repeated regularly (typically at least once a year) to determine if the glaucoma is stable or not. If the visual field progressively gets darker, this can mean that the glaucoma is getting worse, or is more advanced.

Later in this book, we will talk about glaucoma through a lamp analogy, where advancing glaucoma is like the brightness of the lamp's light getting dimmer and dimmer. If the optic nerve gets damaged enough,

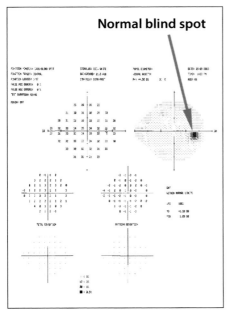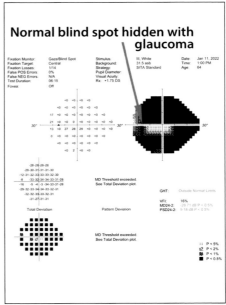

Figure 1.10. Normal (A) and abnormal (B) visual fields.

at the end stage it is like pulling the cord of the lamp out of the wall socket, with the light completely going out. If a person's glaucoma gets worse, then the doctor will typically get more aggressive with treatments to lower the pressure in that eye, perhaps with the use of additional eye drops, light energy/laser treatment, or incisional glaucoma surgery. These efforts help significantly slow the dimming process, so one can continue to see and function.

What About Eye Pressure?

The body naturally makes a fluid inside the eye, called *aqueous humor*. This fluid drains out of the eye through an internal drainage system. The balance between fluid being made and fluid draining out gives the eye a certain eye pressure. Normal eye pressure for a normal optic nerve is 21 millimeters of mercury (mmHg) or less. When there is an imbalance in this process, it could lead to elevated eye pressure. Elevated eye pressure may put stress on the optic nerve and could damage it, causing glaucoma to develop. It was once believed that you must have glaucoma if you have elevated eye pressure. This is not entirely true, however. Not every patient with mildly elevated eye pressure will develop glaucoma when their nerve is healthy. We call these patients *ocular hypertensives*. Although their eye pressure is high, their nerve status and visual field status are still healthy.

Here is a weight-lifter analogy to help you better understand the risk of elevated eye pressure; see figures 1.11 and 1.12. Depending on how high the pressure is and what other risk factors are present (such as status of the nerve, thickness of the cornea, and family history), a doctor may decide to monitor the condition closely, without treatment (fig. 1.13), versus treating the patient to prevent glaucoma development by lowering the eye pressure.

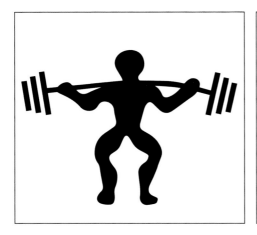

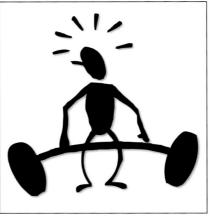

Figure 1.11. For a strong weight lifter—a healthy optic nerve—the pressure of the weight is nicely in balance.

Figure 1.12. A weak weight lifter—a damaged optic nerve—cannot maintain their balance because the pressure of the weight is too much for them.

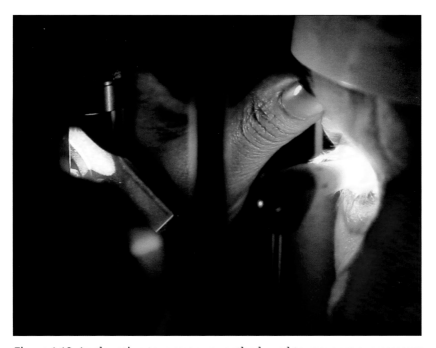

Figure 1.13. Applanation tonometry, a method used to measure eye pressure.

What About When the Pressure Is Not High?

Glaucoma can occur at any pressure level—high, low, or normal. In fact, at least half of the people with glaucoma have normal eye pressures. The problem with glaucoma is really about the damage that occurs to the structure of the nerve and the resulting loss of vision. We know that part of what causes the optic nerve to become damaged is the effect that baseline eye pressure has on the optic nerve. *Baseline pressure* is the eye pressure at the time of a glaucoma diagnosis, before any treatment. If the optic nerve is getting damaged, the eye pressure must come down below the baseline pressure to help slow down the rate of damage. This is the only way in which we know how to manage glaucoma, because other factors are out of our control.

What Is Good Eye Pressure?

If you are diagnosed with glaucoma, you may hear the term *target pressure*. This is a designated eye pressure that your doctor will determine based on your clinical picture. This target pressure is an estimated pressure; maintaining it should slow the rate of nerve damage significantly. A target pressure can remain unchanged if the nerve structure and visual function remain stable over time. If the nerve structure or function (or both) get worse, however, the target pressure may need to be changed. Your treatment regimen will then be altered to reach a new, lower target pressure.

Although there is currently no cure for glaucoma, we know that we can manage the disease by decreasing the eye pressure from its baseline measurement. If done adequately and consistently, this will help slow down the progressive nature of the disease and can continue do so for several years.

Glaucoma Is Sneaky

The major problem with glaucoma is that it typically lacks symptoms. There are several forms of glaucoma. (See the section on "What Are the Types of Glaucoma?" for more detail.) The two most common forms are open-angle and angle-closure glaucoma.

By far the majority of diagnosed glaucoma in the United States is open-angle glaucoma. In the early stages of open-angle glaucoma, you can't tell if you have an eye disease. There isn't a sudden symptom that can alert you to get your eyes checked. The early signs are very subtle and are often ignored. Unfortunately, once the symptoms become significant and noticeable, there is irreversible damage.

Angle-closure glaucoma, compared with open-angle glaucoma, is not diagnosed as frequently in the US, and it occurs more commonly in Asian populations. That being said, angle-closure glaucoma can still occur in all races and is seen readily in the US. The symptoms of angle-closure glaucoma are often not as silent as those for open-angle glaucoma. Common symptoms could show up in the form of a subtle headache or pressure around the eye, often mistaken for a sinus headache. Further, a person with angle-closure glaucoma could have an angle-closure attack, where one can experience sudden intense eye pressure, pain, headache, decreased vision, and eye redness. This is a true eye emergency, and you will need to seek immediate eye care. Permanent vision loss can occur quickly in this setting, and treatment often involves using an eye laser or a surgical procedure, in addition to medical therapy.

Screening Is the Answer

When glaucoma is caught early, it is much easier to treat. This is why getting screened for glaucoma is so vital. The chance of still having a lifetime of good functional vision is high. When someone does have a noticeable loss of vision, however, the damage at that point is usually moderate to severe and cannot be corrected. In that situation, a doctor can only try to preserve the remaining optic nerve tissue and vision. There is hopeful research about glaucoma and the ability to regenerate nerve tissue outside of the body.[1] Nonetheless, no available clinical treatments exist to successfully regrow functional nerve tissue in the eye—at least not yet. One nonprofit organization I collaborate with that is fighting for a cure for glaucoma is the Glaucoma Research Foundation. You can visit their website and gain more information about fighting for a cure at www.glaucoma.org.

What Does Glaucoma Look Like? Part 2

So now that you have a better understanding of what glaucoma is, let's look at another analogy, through the viewpoint of a lamp and light.

Viewpoint 2: The Optic Nerve Is Like a Lamp's Cable Cord

Think of a lamp and how it works. The lamp, like the eye, is made up of individual parts (such as the bulb, socket, neck, base, and shade). They can all be working just fine, but if the cord of the lamp is not plugged in, the lamp won't light.

Similarly, think of the optic nerve as a cable cord between the eye and the brain (fig. 1.14). Signals for vision are sent from the eye to the brain through this optic nerve. If the cable is not functioning fully, the visual ability of the eye will be affected. If the optic nerve is completely damaged, it's like an unplugged lamp. There can be complete loss of vision, to the point of perceiving no light.

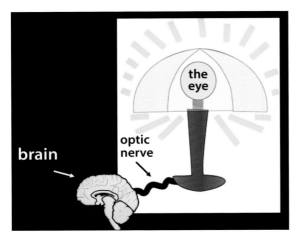

Figure 1.14. A lamp analogy.

Glaucoma is usually a slow process, not a sudden one. You could even lose half of your nerve cells and not begin to notice your glaucoma. The signs are often subtle until the late stages.

Look at the image below with the light bulb (fig. 1.15). At full 100% brightness, this is like a normal healthy nerve. You have plenty of expanded vision to see well and clearly.

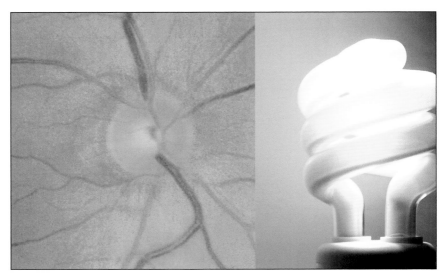

Figure 1.15. An optic nerve (*left*) and light bulb (*right*) at 100% brightness.

If you lost 50% of the nerve tissue, and thus brightness, you would still have light that would enable you to function (fig. 1.16). Your field of vision could very well still be normal. The majority of people at this stage would not notice the change, because it would be gradual.

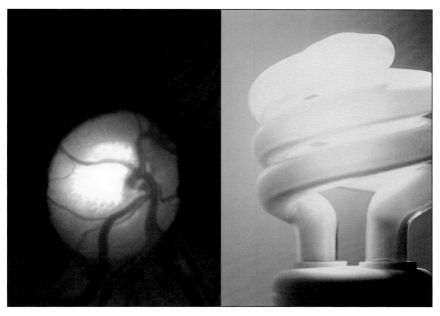

Figure 1.16. An optic nerve (*left*) and lightbulb (*right*) at 50% brightness.

If you lost 70% of your nerve tissue and were down to 30% brightness, you might begin to notice a problem (fig. 1.17). You could probably still function fairly well. Maybe it would take a bit more work to see and accomplish what you were doing before, but you could still do it. You could ignore the signs or attribute them to aging or to being tired. Or you could decide to get checked to see if you need glasses and then find out you have another problem.

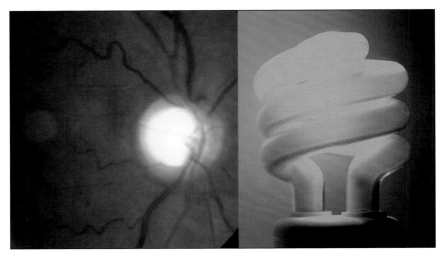

Figure 1.17. An optic nerve (*left*) and light bulb (*right*) at 30% brightness.

If you lost 85% of the nerve tissue and were down to 15% brightness, you would definitely notice signs of a problem (fig. 1.18). This condition will begin to take a toll on your ability to function. At this stage, you have moderate to advanced glaucoma. Treatments are aimed at helping you maintain function and are not a cure. Unfortunately, the currently available treatments cannot completely stop the progression of nerve cell loss. Also, at this later stage, the treatment efforts often need to be more aggressive to have an impact.

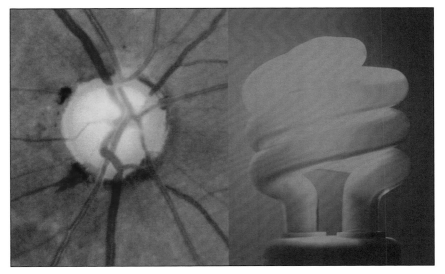

Figure 1.18. An optic nerve (*left*) and light bulb (*right*) at 15% brightness.

If you lost 95% to 99% of the nerve tissue, you would have reached legal blindness (fig. 1.19).

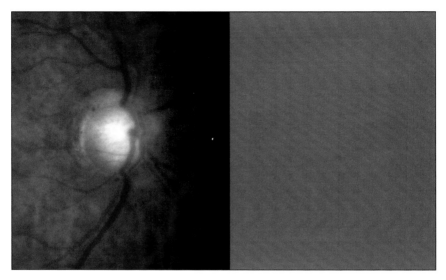

Figure 1.19. An optic nerve (*left*) and light bulb (*right*) at 5% brightness.

I paint this picture not to scare you, but to try to educate you. When you understand what glaucoma can do, you will see why it is crucial to get screened early, and, if diagnosed, to follow up regularly with your eye doctor to preserve your vision.

Also understand that glaucoma is a complex eye disease, and each person with glaucoma may experience vision loss differently. Glaucoma can affect certain areas of the optic nerve specifically (focal loss), or it can affect many areas of the optic nerve generally (global loss). Because of this variability, each person experiences what glaucoma looks like in their own unique way.

What is similar, though, is that if glaucoma is left untreated, it can cause diminished color vision, reduced contrast sensitivity (the ability to tell subtle differences between finer and finer light levels versus full dark), and difficulty with depth perception. It ultimately can lead to complete blindness, a drastic result that we want to prevent through education and action. Keep reading.

What Are the Types of Glaucoma?

We have mentioned that glaucoma is a complex eye disease. As such, there are several types of glaucoma. By far the most common types are open-angle glaucoma and angle-closure glaucoma. The classification of these types is based on the position of certain structures in the eye.

Open-Angle Glaucoma

Within the eye there is a structure called the *ciliary body*. This structure continually creates fluid, or *aqueous humor*, that nourishes the inside of the eye. Aqueous humor flows from the ciliary body around another structure, called the *iris*, into a space called the *anterior chamber*. It then flows out of the eye through a drainage system and gets absorbed into other parts of the body.

The entry point of this drainage system is called the *trabecular meshwork*. When we examine the eye through a special instrument called a *gonioprism*, this lens allows us to see a magnified view of the trabecular meshwork and other structures around it. When these structures look like they are in a normal position and one can see the trabecular meshwork well, we call this an open angle.

What occurs in open-angle glaucoma is that there is some type of clog within the drainage system (fig. 1.20). This clog prevents the aqueous humor from draining well, despite the eye structures appearing normal. It eventually causes an increase in eye pressure due to the back up of fluid drainage. As the increased pressure pushes against the walls of the eye, the pressure causes damage to the delicate fibers of the optic nerve in a permanent way, and thus open-angle glaucoma begins.

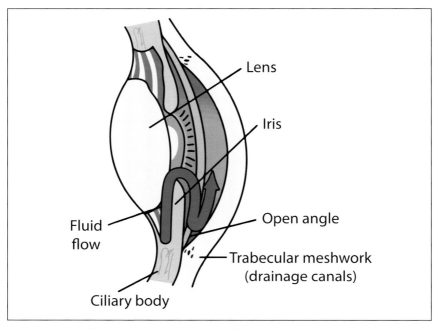

Figure 1.20. Fluid pathway in open-angle glaucoma.

Angle-Closure Glaucoma

In angle-closure glaucoma, the aqueous humor being made from the ciliary body flows in a different pathway to the drainage system, causing pressure behind the iris, which pushes it forward (fig. 1.21). This forward position of the iris results in a blockage of the trabecular meshwork, which further prevents the aqueous humor from flowing out through the trabecular meshwork. We can use a gonioprism to magnify the area and identify angle closure.

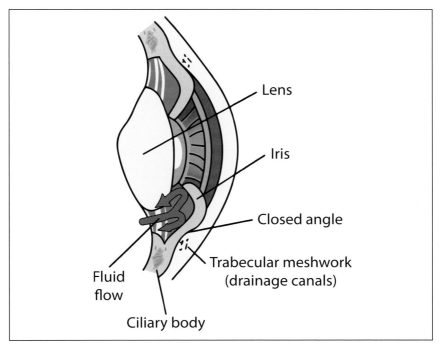

Figure 1.21. Fluid pathway in angle-closure glaucoma.

Glaucoma Is Like a Sink

To understand the difference between open-angle and angle-closure glaucoma, picture a sink with a drain and a running faucet. As mentioned earlier, fluid is continuously made in the eye, which is like a running faucet that is always turned on. There is an internal drainage system in the eye that drains this fluid, like an unclogged, open sink drain (fig. 1.22A). There is a balance between the fluid being made and the fluid going out of the drain, creating normal pressure in the eye.

When a person suffers from open-angle glaucoma, it is like there is a clog inside the drain (fig. 1.22B). The faucet continues to flow, but the fluid can't escape. In a sink, the fluid would eventually build up and spill over the edge of the sink. In the eye, however, the fluid cannot drain out, because it is a closed system. So when the fluid builds up, the pressure increases. This puts stress on the optic nerve, causing damage and, ultimately, worsened open-angle glaucoma.

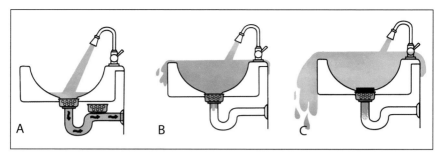

Figure 1.22. Glaucoma sink analogy for (A) a normal eye, (B) primary open-angle glaucoma, and (C) angle-closure glaucoma.

In angle-closure glaucoma, though, the "clog" occurs toward the opening of the drain. It acts as a stopper, preventing the fluid from the faucet from even entering the drain (fig. 1.22C). Angle closure can create extremely high pressure very rapidly. This is a medical emergency that needs to be treated quickly, as severe, irreversible damage to the optic nerve can happen fast.

Other Types of Glaucoma

There are several other types of glaucoma, but a complete discussion of them is beyond the scope of this book. Here we will simply mention them briefly.

Congenital Glaucoma

Congenital glaucoma affects babies and is a result of poor development of the structures in the eye that allow proper fluid drainage. This condition is uncommon. Symptoms can include excess tear production, cloudy or grayish-looking eyes, and eyes that appear larger in size when seen early in infancy. Treatments for this condition are often surgical.

Secondary Glaucoma

This type of glaucoma is a generalized term that can encompass many subsets of glaucoma that are secondary causes of open-angle or angle-closure glaucoma. They can be caused by trauma to the eye, the use of steroids or other medications that can elevate eye pressures, diabetes, inflammation in the eye, the development of a mature cataract, or a tumor. The issue each form of secondary glaucoma has in common is elevated eye pressure, which has a damaging effect on the optic nerve.

Pigment Dispersion Glaucoma
Pigment dispersion glaucoma occurs when there is an extra release of pigment particles from the colored structure in your eye, called the iris. Since these particles have to escape out of the eye through the same drainage system as the aqueous humor, over time the pigment particles can clog the drain and cause eye pressure to rise.

Pseudoexfoliative Glaucoma
In this type of glaucoma, there is a genetic development of protein material that collects in the eye and sloughs off in small pieces over time. Those pieces can get stuck in the drainage system and eventually cause a significant clog that creates elevated eye pressure.

Normal-Tension Glaucoma
Normal-tension glaucoma is a subset of open-angle glaucoma that occurs in patients who have normal to low eye pressure. Damage begins from an unknown problem that shows up as weakness within the optic nerve structure. The nerve can easily be damaged, even with normal or low eye pressure.

Traumatic Glaucoma
This type of glaucoma occurs when there is direct trauma or injury to the eye. Damage to certain structures within the drainage system cause a poor outflow of aqueous humor, and resulting elevation in eye pressure can damage the optic nerve.

Neovascular Glaucoma

Neovascular glaucoma is caused by a vascular problem within the eye that is related to conditions like diabetes or high blood pressure. Here, a signal is turned on in the eye, which creates additional blood vessels that act like weeds, spreading haphazardly and wildly throughout the eye. They can bleed easily, causing inflammation and scarring, which can ultimately clog the drainage system. Eye pressure is then elevated, causing damage to the optic nerve.

Uveitic Glaucoma

This type of glaucoma occurs as a result of inflammation within the eye. The inflammatory cells can clog the drainage system or cause scarring that obstructs it. The treatment for inflammation typically involves steroids, which, in turn, could cause an elevation in eye pressure. The source of the inflammation could be from trauma, a systemic or body condition such as arthritis, or unknown causes.

Steroid-Induced Glaucoma

People with glaucoma commonly have elevated eye pressure related to their use of steroids. That usage could be in the form of topical steroid drops in the eye; inhaled steroids, such as from devices to treat breathing problems; topical steroid ointments for skin conditions; steroid injections, such as for damaged knee joints; or oral steroids. It is important for those using steroids for chronic conditions or at high doses to be checked for eye pressure elevation.

How Is Glaucoma Diagnosed?

Look closely at this picture of three eyes (fig. 1.23). Which of these eyes has glaucoma?

Any or none of these eyes could have glaucoma. Your guess would be as good as mine. The reality is that looking at someone's eye from the outside, you can't tell that glaucoma lies within. This is why regular eye screening is so important.

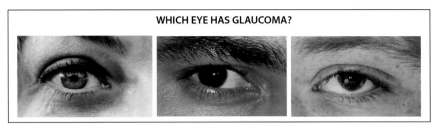

Figure 1.23. Eyes that could potentially have glaucoma.

In order to diagnose someone with glaucoma, a thorough eye examination in a clinical setting is required. There are multiple tests performed during an eye exam in order to decide whether glaucoma is present.

Tests for Glaucoma

Vision Test

Checking the *visual acuity* of each eye measures how good your vision is. This test is typically performed by looking off in the distance at a chart that has various letters or shapes in different sizes (fig. 1.24). By finding out how much of the chart you can read, the doctor can assess how healthy your vision is in each eye. Perfect vision is considered to be 20/20—in other words, your eye can see what is expected for normal healthy vision at a distance of 20 feet.

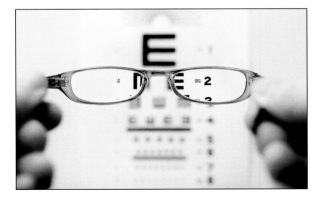

Figure 1.24. Looking at a vision chart.

Slit-Lamp Exam

A *slit lamp* is a common tool used to evaluate the eye (fig. 1.25). It has a microscope and special light that allows a doctor to examine your eye in great detail. With special lenses, your doctor also has the ability to look inside your eye and study various structures, such as the optic nerve and retina, to check for any damage.

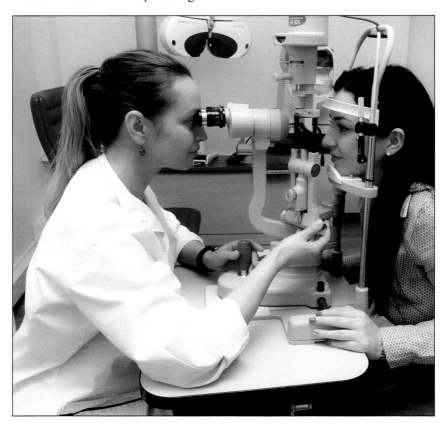

Figure 1.25. A patient being examined with a slit lamp.

Eye Pressure

A process called *tonometry* measures eye pressure. This is typically per-formed after a numbing drop has been placed in the eye. A machine is then used to measure the eye pressure by gently touching the numbed surface of your eye, called the *cornea* (fig. 1.26). There are several different techniques and devices that can determine eye pressure.

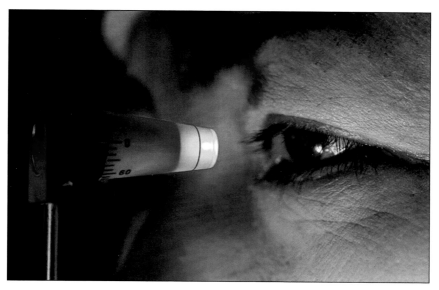

Figure 1.26. Eye pressure being taken with a device called an applanation tonometer.

Gonioscopy

Gonioscopy evaluates the structures in the eye, allowing your doctor to assess your natural drainage system. After a numbing eye drop has been placed in the eye, the procedure is performed with the help of a special lens that makes gentle contact with the surface of your eye (fig. 1.27). The area in the eye that the doctor examines is often referred to as the *angle*, and this is used to define the type of glaucoma one has: either open-angle or closed-angle (narrow) glaucoma.

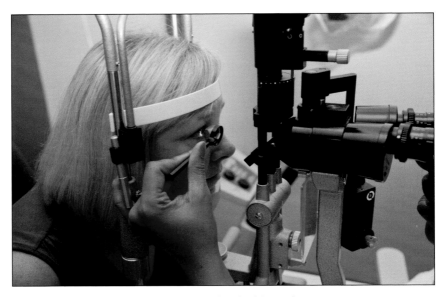

Figure 1.27. A patient's eye being examined with gonioscopy.

Visual Field Test

A visual field test is also called *perimetry*. This is a test of your side, or peripheral, vision and can tell the doctor if your vision has been affected by glaucoma (fig. 1.28). If you have glaucoma, this test will be repeated many times to evaluate if your glaucoma is stable. There is a learning curve with the test, meaning that as you take repeated tests in the future, you get better and more accurate each time. This can be a frustrating test for some because it evaluates areas where you can see as well as areas where you can't, which can make it feel as if you are not doing well while you complete the test. Just make sure that you are well rested before taking the test and try to do your best.

Nerve Fiber Layer Analysis

There are various types of imaging tests of the optic nerve that can help examine it in great detail. The most common is called *OCT*, or *optical coherence tomography*. It can give a direct measure of the thickness of the nerve fiber layer and, over time, help your doctor assess whether

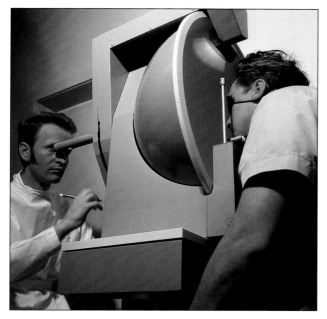

Figure 1.28. A patient taking a visual field test.

damage to the optic nerve is stable or progressively getting worse. In figure 1.29, the green color indicates healthy nerve tissue, yellow indicates borderline healthy nerve tissue, and red indicates severe damage.

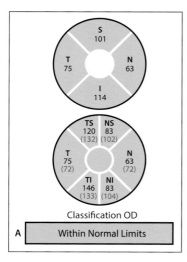

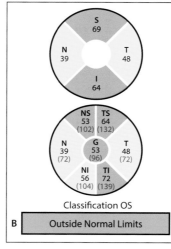

Figure 1.29. Optical coherence tomography diagnostic tests: (A) normal; (B) abnormal.

Photographs of the Optic Nerve

A picture is worth a thousand words. Photographs of the optic nerve allow your doctor to have a record of how the nerve looks at one point in time, so it can be compared with future views of the nerve to assess any changes (fig. 1.30). This test is often done when the eyes are dilated.

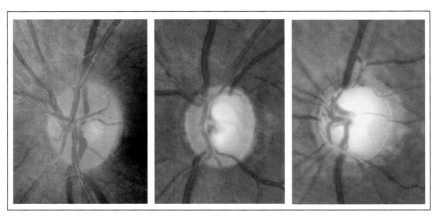

Figure 1.30. Optic nerve photographs taken at various stages of severity.

Test Results

After these tests are performed and the results are reviewed by your eye doctor, a diagnosis of glaucoma, as well as a determination of the type of glaucoma and its stage (mild, moderate, or severe), should be able to be made. At times the presence of glaucoma is not definite, but suspected. A patient in this scenario is then given a diagnosis of *glaucoma suspect*. There may be no immediate treatment, but that person will undergo continued observation and repeated tests. Let's next talk about the treatment options for glaucoma.

How Is Glaucoma Treated?

Whether the glaucoma is open angle or angle closure, and is mild, moderate or severe, all treatment methods are aimed at the same goal: to lower the baseline eye pressure. Think of eye pressure like stress on the optic nerve. If one can reduce the stress, this can protect the remaining optic nerve tissue and prevent further damage, as well as a possible permanent loss of vision.

The three pillars of treatment for glaucoma are medications, light energy (laser) treatment, and incisional surgery. Medications are still the most commonly used treatment method for glaucoma, though there has been a more recent shift to utilizing light energy or surgical interventions earlier in the process. You may benefit from one type of treatment or several in combination to manage your glaucoma over your lifetime. The various treatment options will be presented to you, and recommendations will be made by your doctor.

Medication

Medications for glaucoma can be taken in the form of eye drops (most common), oral pills, through an IV (an intravenous route), or other modes of sustained-release delivery. There are currently six classes of glaucoma medications, with various generic and brand names. Each class comes in the form of eye drops that have a specific bottle top color, which helps to more easily communicate medication regimens between doctor and patient. This is especially helpful due to some of the complicated names of these drops or complex schedules of usage.

Each medication has potential side effects, which are important to keep in mind when deciding which medication will be the best option for the patient. Also, each medication has a specific mechanism of action for how it lowers eye pressure, which can be additive when multiple medications are used in combination. Let's go over the six different glaucoma drug classes (fig. 1.31).

Class—COLOR OF BOTTLE TOP—Mechanism of Action—Most Common Side Effects

Alpha Agonists—PURPLE TOP—decreases the production of intraocular fluid (aqueous humor) and increases the drainage of the fluid—burning or stinging in the eye, drowsiness, dry mouth and nose, headache, fatigue

Beta Blockers—YELLOW TOP—decreases the production of intraocular fluid—burning or stinging in the eye, reduced pulse rate, lower blood pressure, shortness of breath in people with asthma or breathing disorders, depression, reduced libido

Carbonic Ahhydrase Inhibitors—ORANGE TOP—decreases the production of intraocular fluid—blurred vision, dry eyes, stinging, burning in the eye (side effects of the oral pill in this class includes fatigue, frequent urination, tingling in the hands and feet, upset stomach, kidney stones)

Cholinergics—GREEN TOP—increases the drainage of intraocular fluid—dim vision, headache around the eyebrow, small pupil size

Prostaglandin Analogs—TEAL TOP—increases the drainage of intraocular fluid—red eyes, eye color change in the iris, darkened eyelid skin, eyelash growth, stinging, itching in the eye, dry eyes, sunken eyes

Rho Kinase Inhibitors—WHITE TOP—increases the drainage of intraocular fluid—red eyes, stinging in the eye, pigmentation on the cornea, small amounts of bleeding in the white of the eye

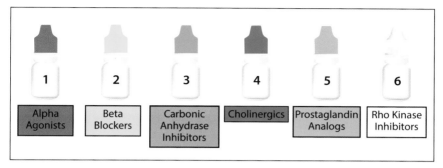

Figure 1.31. Six classes of eye drops and their bottle cap colors.

Of the medication classes listed above, only the carbonic anhydrase inhibitors come in an oral pill form, which can also be given intravenously.

Several classes of drops can come in a combined form in one bottle, for more convenient use and greater potency.

Outside of medications in the form of drops, one class of drug—the prostaglandin analogs—now comes in the form of a sustained-release pellet that can be placed in the eye and help lower eye pressure for a period of months to years.

We are hoping for additional methods of drugs being delivered to the eye, which are in the testing phases now.

Look in the "Resources" section in the back of this book to learn how to properly instill eye drops and how *not* to put them in.

Light Energy (Laser)

We have several different types of light energy treatments. They come in the form of various lasers that can be applied to the eye and effectively lower eye pressure. Which laser is utilized depends on the type of glaucoma and the severity of the condition. These treatments use different wavelengths of light and are aimed at various structures in the eye. Some treatments use a numbing eye drop, with the patient sitting upright in an office setting, while others take place in an operating room, under sterile conditions and with sedation.

Laser Peripheral Iridotomy (LPI)

This laser treatment is used for angle-closure glaucoma. It helps move the obstruction in the drainage system by making a small hole in the iris tissue with a heated laser, so fluid can flow in a different direction. This change in direction helps open up the obstruction. LPI is typically performed in an office setting, with the patient sitting upright, and uses a topical eye drop for anesthesia.

Selective Laser Trabeculoplasty (SLT)

This laser treatment is used for open-angle glaucoma. It helps open the pores of the drainage system within the trabecular meshwork by using a cold laser (fig. 1.32). Because the surrounding tissues are left intact, this procedure can safely be repeated multiple times. SLT is typically performed in the office setting, with the patient sitting upright, and uses a topical eye drop for anesthesia.

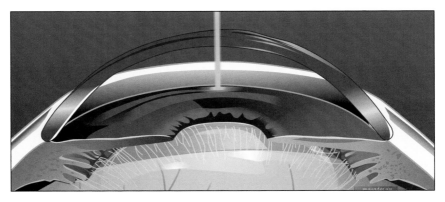

Figure 1.32. SLT light treatment.

Argon Laser Trabeculoplasty (ALT)

This laser treatment is used for open-angle glaucoma. It uses a heated laser to help make the drainage system flow better within the trabecular meshwork. The laser can cause scarring of the tissue within the drainage system, so this type of treatment can't be repeated. ALT is typically performed in an office setting, with the patient sitting upright, and uses a topical eye drop for anesthesia.

Laser Cyclophotocoagulation

This laser treatment is used for open-angle or angle-closure glaucoma. The laser's energy is aimed at a structure called the ciliary body, which makes fluid in the eye. The laser effectively reduces the amount of fluid being created, thus reducing the amount of fluid that needs to be drained, which in turn lowers eye pressure. There are several different methods for how this treatment can be applied to the eye. It could be performed in the procedure room of an office setting or in a sterile operating room, but more numbing of the eye than just drops is required.

Treatment Choices

Studies have shown that laser peripheral iridotomy for angle-closure glaucoma, and selective laser trabeculoplasty for open-angle glaucoma, can be effective first-line therapies.

Incisional Surgery

There are several different types of glaucoma surgery options that can be performed for the various types and stages of glaucoma. A determination of which option is best for a patient can be made at the time of the examination and depends on both the specific glaucoma condition and the skill set and comfort level of the doctor performing the surgery.

Traditional glaucoma surgeries have been available for several decades and are able to lower eye pressure effectively. The most commonly utilized ones are trabeculectomy and a tube shunt. Though these surgeries help lower eye pressure, they can also be associated with some complications that can affect one's vision, and they have a longer healing time. Nonetheless, they are the go-to procedures when glaucoma is more advanced or refractory (meaning it is very difficult to control).

Trabeculectomy

Trabeculectomy is considered the gold standard for glaucoma surgery. In this procedure, incisions are made in the eye to create a new pathway for fluid to flow internally. A *bleb* is created as result of this procedure.

This is a space for intraocular fluid to flow into that can allow the fluid to be absorbed, thus lowering the overall pressure inside the eye. This outpatient procedure is done in an operating room and can take 6 to 8 weeks to heal.

Tube Shunt

In a tube shunt procedure, a device is permanently placed in the eye and acts as a new drainage system. The device can vary in shape and size, but it typically sits along the wall of the eye in an area that is covered by the eyelid. As fluid flows into the tube, it is shunted away to another place internally where it can be absorbed. This reduces overall eye pressure. This outpatient procedure is done in an operating room and can take 6 to 8 weeks to heal.

If you have had a traditional glaucoma procedure, know that there can be risks of infection even years or decades after the surgery has been done. You should alert your doctor if you develop a painful red eye.

MIGS

Minimally invasive glaucoma surgery, or MIGS, is a more recent class of glaucoma surgery. It was developed in order to find solutions to effectively lower eye pressure while reducing some of the risks involved with traditional glaucoma surgery. Though these procedures can reduce eye pressure, they typically are not able to lower them to the level obtained through traditional glaucoma surgeries, so they are often utilized in patients who have mild to moderate glaucoma.

Treatment Choices

These surgical procedures have various mechanisms for how they work, but collectively their goal is to enhance the eye's natural drainage system by clearing away clogged material or using an implanted device within the natural drain to create a stable pathway for intraocular fluid to flow better. Better flow means lower eye pressure. Often these procedures can benefit patients by also reducing the number of eye drops that are needed to help control their glaucoma. Any of these procedures can be done at the same time as cataract surgery, and some can be performed alone. MIGS are outpatient procedure that are done in an operating room and can typically take 4 to 6 weeks to heal.

Who Is at Risk for Glaucoma?

Not everyone will develop glaucoma, but anyone can be at risk. It can occur at any age, for any gender, and in any ethnicity. There are, however, risk factors that make certain people more susceptible to glaucoma than others. Some risk factors are easily discernible by an average person, while others are found through an actual eye exam. Because the list is extensive, we will discuss just some of the most common and important risk factors.

Increasing Age

The risk of glaucoma increases with age. This is because we naturally lose optic nerve tissue as we age. The older you are, the higher the chance that this loss of optic nerve tissue can negatively affect your vision. We can use a jar of marbles as an analogy to illustrate this concept. When we are born, we have a jar full of marbles (fig. 1.33). Each day, we lose about 1 marble. As we get older, the jar gets less full, and we continue to lose marbles at a higher rate. Older people without glaucoma may lose 5 marbles a day. Their jar is half full. They don't have vision loss yet, but we should monitor them closely anyway and begin treatment to slow down the rate of marble loss if they are losing marbles at

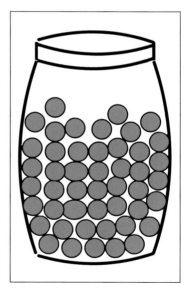

Figure 1.33. A jar of marbles representing an optic nerve.

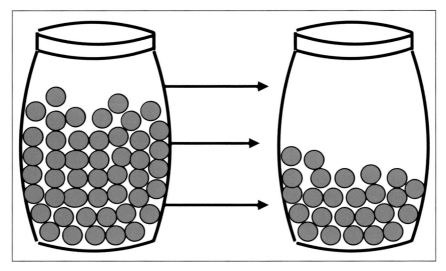

Figure 1.34. Jars of marbles representing a normal optic nerve (*left*) and a weakening optic nerve (*right*).

a much higher rate than normal. Even more elderly people with glaucoma may lose 10 marbles a day. Their jar is only one-fourth full (fig. 1.34). This puts them at a greater risk of vision loss. We should monitor them even more closely and treat them more aggressively.

Family History

If you have glaucoma, anyone who is a blood relative has an increased risk for developing glaucoma. This is especially true for your immediate family, including your siblings, parents, and children. *The rate of glaucoma can be up to nine times higher among individuals with a sibling who has glaucoma.* See Tip 9 (in chapter 2) for further discussion on this topic.

Ethnicity

There are certain ethnicities that are more predisposed to various types of glaucoma.

African or Caribbean Descent

According to many population-based studies, more African Americans have glaucoma, compared with Caucasians. Blindness from glaucoma is 6 to 8 times more common in African Americans than Caucasians.[2] And African Americans are 15 times more likely to be visually impaired from glaucoma than Caucasians.[3] Worldwide, one of the continents at highest risk for blindness from glaucoma is Africa.

Asian Descent

Angle-closure glaucoma is more common in people of Asian descent. People with acute angle-closure glaucoma can have it show up as pain, sensitivity to light, redness in the eyes, and sudden blurred vision. This is a more aggressive form of glaucoma. It makes up less than 10% of the glaucoma diagnosed in the US, but it is much more commonly seen in Asian countries. Angle-closure glaucoma accounts for 90% of all cases of blindness from glaucoma in China.

Another type of glaucoma is called normal-tension glaucoma, where damage to the optic nerve happens when eye pressures are normal or even low. This form of glaucoma seems to occur more commonly in Japanese populations.[4]

Hispanic Descent

Glaucoma is also more common in Hispanic populations, especially in those with predominantly European ancestry. A population-based study showed the overall prevalence of open-angle glaucoma among Hispanics to be nearly 5%, similar to that for those of African descent.[5] This and other studies also indicate that as Hispanics age, the incidence of glaucoma increases exponentially for those over the age of 60.[6]

Scandinavian Descent

Pseudoexfoliative glaucoma tends to occur more commonly in people of Scandinavian descent. This type of glaucoma is associated with the production of a certain type of protein that collects in various parts of the body. In the eye, it can be seen as a fluffy white material that collects on the iris and the lens (fig. 1.35). It can cause an aggressive type of glaucoma and makes cataract removal during surgery more difficult.

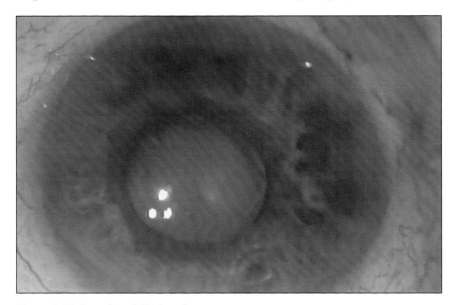

Figure 1.35. Pseudoexfoliative glaucoma.

Overall Susceptibility

Please note that though some ethnicities may be more predisposed to certain types of glaucoma, this doesn't mean that they cannot get other types of glaucoma. Each type of glaucoma can affect any race, gender, or nationality.

Trauma

An injury to the eye or the structure around the eye can increase the risk of glaucoma, although glaucoma as a result of trauma usually occurs only in the injured eye. It may be present immediately after the injury, or it can take several months or even years to develop. Not all people with a history of an eye injury will develop glaucoma. It does put you at a higher risk, however, and should prompt the need for an eye exam soon after the trauma occurs.

Use of Steroids

Steroids are a class of drugs used to treat inflammation in the body. These are different from the anabolic steroids that athletes might use. Steroids can be prescribed in many forms, such as in eye drops, oral pills, injections, an inhaled treatment, and a topical cream. Steroids are used for a variety of reasons. Taking steroids may lead to elevated eye pressure and eventual glaucoma. It is very important to schedule regular follow-up exams with your eye doctor to check your eye pressure if you are using steroid eye drops or steroids for other parts of the body for a longer period of time.

Myopia, or Nearsightedness

If you are nearsighted, you typically can see well up close but can't see distant objects clearly. This is called myopia. It commonly occurs when the eyeball is too long, so light is focused too far in front of the information-processing center of the eye. Population-based studies show that the risk of glaucoma is higher with an increasing degree of nearsightedness.[7,8] This means that the longer your eyeball is, the higher the chance that you will have damage to your optic nerve, and the more likely it is that you will have glaucoma.

Blood Pressure

High blood pressure does not have a direct relationship with an increase in eye pressure, but there can be an indirect relationship, which could have an impact on the development of glaucoma. If you have elevated blood pressure, you should have regular eye screenings.

Low blood pressure can be a problem for glaucoma patients, because it is important for the optic nerve to receive an adequate amount of blood flow to be well nourished. Limited blood flow has been associated with optic nerve damage and is a risk factor for the development of glaucoma.

It is important to tell your eye doctor if you have high or low blood pressure, particularly if you are taking medications for the condition. Some blood pressure medications can affect your glaucoma treatment, so be sure to share this information as well.

Recommendations for Eye Exams

For patients who do not have risk factors for glaucoma, the American Academy of Ophthalmology recommends comprehensive eye exams (table 1.1).

TABLE 1.1. AMERICAN ACADEMY OF OPHTHALMOLOGY EXAM RECOMMENDATIONS FOR PEOPLE WITH NO GLAUCOMA RISK FACTORS

Under 40 years old	every 5–10 years
40–54 years old	every 2–4 years
55–64 years old	every 1–3 years
65 years and older	every 1–2 years

Source: Adapted from Preferred Practice Patterns: Comprehensive Adult Medical Eye Evaluation, American Academy of Ophthalmology, 2022.

A comprehensive eye exam includes

- a detailed evaluation of your medical and eye history,

- a review of your medications,

- an eye health evaluation, including a dilated eye exam,

- measurement of your eye pressure,

- a test of your visual ability, and

- possibly additional tests, depending on the initial findings.

As you get older, you should get comprehensive eye exams more often. If you have additional risk factors for glaucoma (keep reading to find out more about these), eye evaluation should begin even earlier (table 1.2).

TABLE 1.2. AMERICAN ACADEMY OF OPHTHALMOLOGY EXAM RECOMMENDATIONS FOR PEOPLE WITH GLAUCOMA RISK FACTORS

Under 40 years old	every 1–2 years
40–54 years old	every 1–3 years
55 years and older	every 1–2 years

Source: Adapted from Preferred Practice Patterns: Comprehensive Adult Medical Eye Evaluation, American Academy of Ophthalmology, 2015.

What Is the Impact of Glaucoma?

Worldwide, glaucoma is the leading cause of irreversible blindness. Many people do not realize they have glaucoma because vision loss typically is subtle and unnoticeable until the disease is more advanced. In the United States, up to 50% of the people who actually have glaucoma right now do not realize they have it.[9] That number reaches 90% on the global scale. Worldwide, as of 2040, an estimated 80 million people will have been diagnosed with glaucoma.[10] In the US, more than 120,000 are blind from glaucoma, accounting for 9% to 12% of all cases of blindness.[11]

As our aging population continues to grow, the number of people with glaucoma will continue to rise. In the US right now, there are about 3.5 million people with glaucoma, at a cost of approximately $5.8 billion per year from more than 10 million physician visits annually.[12] By 2050, that number will double, with an estimated 7.32 million people having primary open-angle glaucoma.[13]

Although the onset of glaucoma in our populations is on the rise (fig. 1.36), the good news is that the negative impacts of glaucoma in stealing one's vision can be lessened with awareness and by taking personal action. In the next pages I will share some of my top tips that will arm you with clear directions on how to preserve your sight.

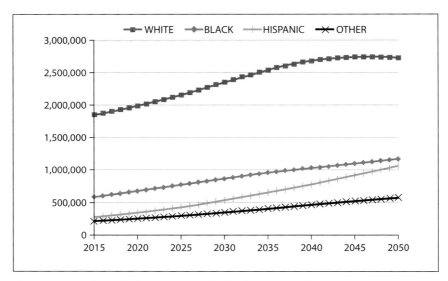

Figure 1.36. Projected glaucoma population by race and year.
Source: Courtesy of Prevent Blindness

2

12 Expert Tips to Prevent Blindness

TIP 1. DON'T IGNORE THE SIGNS

It is true that in the early stages of glaucoma there are minimal, if any, signs. I found that my own patients with moderate to advanced glaucoma, however, ignored many signs of vision changes several years prior to seeing me. These signs were written off as "just my imagination" or "just the process of getting older." My advice to you is to become more cognizant of any visual changes in your regular daily life. If these changes occur, do yourself a favor and get your eyes checked. Time could be of the essence.

Scenario #1: Love of Basketball

One of my patients was a skilled basketball player. As a point guard, he prided himself on seeing everything that was happening on the court to aid in his ability to pass. About 7 years prior to his glaucoma diagnosis, he began to notice that his accuracy in passing and receiving passes was way off. Others noticed this as well. He thought aging was decreasing his skill set. He eventually felt playing basketball was too much effort and not as much fun, so he gave it up. Little did he know that the major reason for this inaccuracy was his gradual peripheral vision loss from glaucoma.

Scenario #2: Scared When Driving with a Child

Another one of my patients loved driving. He would have no problem driving long distances, or driving at night without glasses. About 5 years prior to his diagnosis, he realized that he had to look around a whole lot more than he used to. It was getting harder to drive, because he didn't trust his vision as he once did. One rainy night, when he had to pick up his child from basketball practice, he realized he could not drive safely due to his poor vision (fig. 2.1). He was sweating the whole way home, because he was afraid of putting his child in danger. Even though he had known family members who were losing or had

Figure 2.1. Blurred vision in the rain.

lost vision from glaucoma, it still took what seemed like a near-death experience for him to understand the importance of getting screened.

Other patients have told me that they bump into things more often (for example, hitting the curb when driving or striking the car's side mirror because of faulty judgment). Some report that things just come up on them quickly, whether while driving or being approached by a person.

Don't assume that these types of events are just the result of old age. We have seen significant advances in technology today, and many diseases are treatable and preventable. Don't assume everything that happens visually is simply because you are getting older. Let someone look at your eyes. Chances are, there is some level of treatment for improvement, or to reduce the pace of worsening eyesight.

TIP 2. DO THE "COVER YOUR EYES SO YOU CAN SEE" TEST

With both eyes open, our brain processes information from both eyes to give us the best possible vision. When one eye cannot see well, the other can compensate. I have seen countless times when patients have a significant reduction of vision in one eye but, frankly, never noticed it until someone asked them in a clinical exam to cover the good eye. Because of this, a significant visual deficit can go unnoticed if a person doesn't check each eye individually.

Disclaimer: This is a test that is NOT specific for glaucoma. Any eye condition that is vision-threatening can create a positive test. Moreover, if your test is normal, this does NOT mean that you do not have glaucoma. Only an eye care professional would be able to determine that. This test is no substitute for an in-person eye examination, which is recommended for glaucoma screening. It is simply a useful tool to prompt an eye exam that can further diagnose a problem.

How to Do the Test

When you cover one eye and look out the uncovered eye, you can evaluate your vision in that particular eye (fig. 2.2).

1. Take time to notice both your central vision (clarity when looking straight ahead) and peripheral vision (the ability to see what is to the side of you without looking directly at it). If you have been prescribed glasses or contact lenses, the test should be done with your corrective eyewear in place.

2. Cover one eye and look out the uncovered eye. Can you still see clearly?

3. Cover the opposite eye and look out the uncovered eye. Can you still see clearly? How does it compare with the first eye?

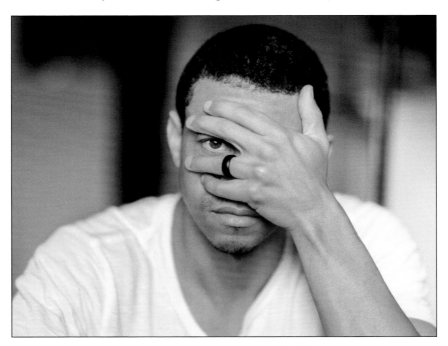

Figure 2.2. A man covering one of his eyes to test his vision.

This test helps you discover if there are significant disparities between the vision in each of your eyes. If you notice a significant difference between how well you see in steps 2 and 3, you should contact an eye care specialist promptly. This may save your vision. Try this test now!

TIP 3. ACCEPT THE DISEASE, DON'T ACCEPT DEFEAT

If you have been told you have glaucoma, the initial shock of the diagnosis can feel very unreal. This is understandable, especially if you are still seeing well and functioning normally. It is very easy to want to feel fine and, thus, go into a state of denial. This denial also can be present when you are told you have a high risk for developing glaucoma, either because of how your eyes look or because you have a blood relative known to have the disease. If you stay in denial or are fearful of finding out that glaucoma may truly be present in your eyes, this actually prevents you from being your own advocate to protect the precious sight you do have.

Remember, accepting that you have glaucoma does not mean that you have to accept defeat in what seems like an incurable situation. Don't fall into feeling like a victim, because that mindset can make it hard to empower yourself to take actions that can keep you seeing better longer. Also, don't be afraid to accept support or help from your family (fig. 2.3).

Here are some ways to better manage a glaucoma diagnosis:

• Accept the disease. When you have been diagnosed with glaucoma by a trusted doctor, your glaucoma doesn't go away, and it won't go on pause, just because you're not ready to accept it. Staying in denial will not help slow down the disease. If you're able to accept the disease now, you can actually take control of it and do something about it. You have to be your own advocate.

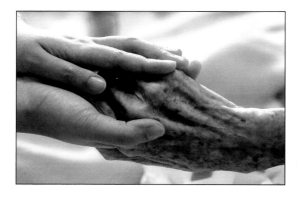

Figure 2.3. Accepting
family help.

• Accept the risk that you can lose vision from glaucoma, so you can take the necessary action to keep seeing.

• When in doubt, get a second or even a third opinion from a glaucoma specialist. Look at the "Resources" section the back of this book for a guide on how to find a glaucoma specialist.

• Accept that you have the power to control the best possible outcome for your sight.

TIP 4. CONQUER YOUR FEARS: DON'T DESPAIR, HAVE HOPE

Glaucoma is an eye disease that typically doesn't have symptoms in its early stages. It is called the "silent thief of sight" for this reason. Therefore, it's important to be screened early, when simpler treatment strategies are most effective. This is especially true for those at highest risk.

Once you accept that you have glaucoma, you can be an advocate for your vision. Remember the following pieces of advice:

1. *Glaucoma can lead to blindness, but don't despair!* Most patients do not go blind from glaucoma if they get treatment for it.

2. *Treatment aimed at lowering eye pressure does work to prevent vision loss.* Find a doctor who you can trust (see Tip 6 on "Partnering with Your Doctor").

3. *Conquer your fears.* Glaucoma can be a disease where people feel very alone and isolated, because they feel that the world does not understand what they are seeing through their eyes. But you don't have to go through this alone. When you talk to other patients who have glaucoma, you realize that you are not alone. You can gain information on things others have done that have helped them, and that you can do, too. You can also share your story and feel empowered by helping someone else. Support groups could be found in places as simple as the waiting area of your doctor's office. I know many of my patients with glaucoma talk to each other while waiting for their eye exam, often finding support and encouragement by sharing their stories with each other. To find other support groups that meet in person, you can check with hospitals and eye care centers in your area. Facebook and Yahoo have online groups for glaucoma who can offer help. Also, don't forget about sharing with your family. They can often be a huge area for support if you open up to them on what you are going through and need help with.

4. *Have hope!* We are in exciting times for glaucoma. Many new medications, new ways of delivering medications, and new, less invasive surgical techniques are coming out now. Have hope that help is available now and that more is to come in the future (fig. 2.4).

5. *If you currently have some visual impairment from glaucoma, I strongly encouraged you to seek help through vision rehabilitation services, which can maximize your health, quality of life, and independence.* This process begins with a referral to a low-vision optometric specialist, followed by a visual efficiency and function evaluation, and then specified care. During this exam, the specialist will find out what your limitations are—that is, what specific activities you may be

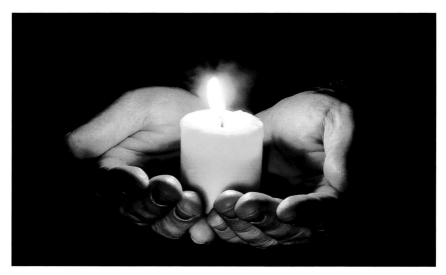

Figure 2.4. Hands holding a candle of hope.

having trouble with—so they can find tools to help. This could be as simple as a magnifying glass. There are many different types of magnifiers, and finding the best one for a specific task can make all the difference in the world. The specialist can also offer suggestions and advice on other topics, such as proper lighting, or the importance of creating more contrast to see better in your home or the environment you are in. Overall, the goal of treatment is to enable you to do all the things you did before you lost vision, with help and the resources to do them in a different—but effective—way.

To find additional helpful resources for you and your loved ones related to the diagnosis of glaucoma, look at the "Resources" section in the back of this book.

TIP 5. TAKE GLAUCOMA SERIOUSLY

Take your glaucoma diagnosis seriously. Although you may want to take a break from the recommended treatment regimen or follow-ups, glaucoma doesn't take breaks. Glaucoma can be progressive, aggressive, and relentless. It is vital that you:

- Follow your eye doctor's recommendations.
  - ~ If you have questions or concerns, speak up and talk your doctor about them.

- Return for scheduled visits appropriately.
  - ~If your appointment gets cancelled and is not rescheduled, call and make a follow-up appointment. You need to be seen regularly.

- Take an active role in your disease.
  - ~ Learn as much as you can to help you live best with your glaucoma.

- Visit the "Resources" section in the back of this book to learn more.

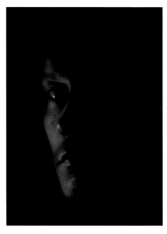

Figure 2.5. A diagnosis of glaucoma should be taken seriously.

When you do this, you are your best advocate to help prevent vision loss.

TIP 6. PARTNERING WITH YOUR DOCTOR

Glaucoma is a chronic eye disease that, once diagnosed, will be lifelong. In order to prevent vision loss, it needs to be treated. Though you play a major role in advocating for your best vision, your eye doctor is your partner in doing this effectively.

Good glaucoma care should start with confidence in your doctor. This is extremely important, because you will be receiving advice and recommendations from your doctor that you should be able to take and adhere to. If confidence is not there, you—as the patient—may not do what is recommended, which could be detrimental to your vision.

This confidence often stems from good doctor-patient rapport, where you feel like you are being listened to. Doctors should be able to listen to your concerns and questions, so they can provide solutions to those problems, as well as give you reassurance and a feeling that there is a good plan in place to help your preserve your vision.

Effective strategies for working with your doctor include keeping track of your appointments. Follow-up care is vital in maintaining control of glaucoma—that is, being able to assess if there is a problem or if things are stable. As you prepare for your eye appointment, it's important to make a list of questions or concerns that came up during the months since your previous doctor's visit, and to consider whether you need refills on your medications. Review this list when you are with your doctor to get those questions or concerns answered and to obtain any necessary prescriptions.

It's also important to be very open and honest with your doctor. As a patient, you want to please the doctor and make sure you do what you are told. But we all know that life happens, and sometimes there are issues related to the treatment that we, as doctors, need to know about so we can come up with a better plan or solution for you. Maybe your medications cause irritation in your eye or other symptoms that make you not want to use your drops. Maybe the medication is so expensive that you can't afford it, so you don't get it, or you try to stretch out the timing of when you apply the drops, which is not an effective treatment for you, either. Or maybe the treatment regimen is just too much, and you are unable to keep up with it. All of these things are important for your doctor to know about, so he or she can address these issues and come up with possible solutions for them. Typically, there are multiple other options that can be chosen.

It is important to understand what is going on with your eyes. We know that all the medical words can sound confusing, or even like a foreign language. Your doctor should present you with information about the condition of your eyes in simple terms, as well as clearly explain the treatment options.

Remember, however, that it's essential for you to ask questions. Sometimes you may wonder what is a good question to ask. *Any* question is a good question when you are trying to learn more about how to take care of your eyes.

Here are some common questions YOU should be able to ask and then gain understanding from the answers:

- What is glaucoma?

- Do I or do I NOT have glaucoma?
  - If no (you don't have glaucoma), what is my risk level for getting glaucoma? How often should I return for re-examinations?
  - If yes (you do have glaucoma)

    –What kind of glaucoma do I have?

    –What stage of glaucoma is present in my eyes (mild, moderate, or severe)?

    –What is my eye pressure, and what target pressure is suitable for my eyes?

    –At the end of every eye exam, find out if your eye pressure is on target and whether your glaucoma is stable.

    –If you take eye drops for treatment, you should know which kind of drops to take for glaucoma, as well as their common side effects.

These questions can change over the course of time as things progress.

Overall, you should know what you have to do to maintain and pre-

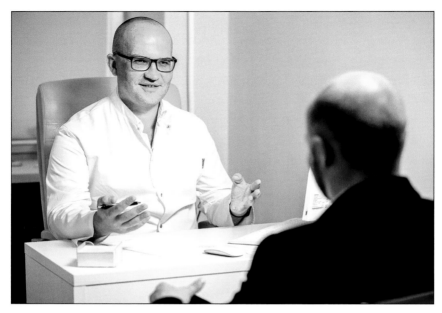

Figure 2.6. A doctor in conversation with a patient.

serve your vision. It is important that you have relevant information about your eyes from a qualified eye care specialist that you can trust and partner with. Write down your questions, so you can go through them one by one with your doctor. Always remember to ask questions and never be afraid (fig. 2.6). The more you know, the more able you are to maintain healthy eyes and preserve your vision.

TIP 7. KNOW WHAT IS EXPECTED

Initial Visits

When you are initially diagnosed with glaucoma, the state of your optic nerve becomes a baseline for an eye doctor to follow over time. This means that he or she will use the image(s) of your optic nerve and compare them with any future ones, looking for any changes. Your eye doctor will document the optic nerve structures by describing them with words, drawing a picture, and probably taking a photograph. A picture is worth a thousand words.

Some of the most common tests include:

- Vision

- Slit lamp exam

- Eye pressure

- Gonioscopy

- Visual field test

- Nerve fiber layer analysis

- Photographs of the optic nerve

Establishing these baseline tests will provide valuable information to see if there is a change in the optic nerve over time.

Repeated Visits

Normally, patients return every 3 to 4 months for checkups. If your glaucoma is mild or stable, you can return every 6 months to a year. If you have recently had glaucoma surgery, however, or if your treatment regimen is still being established, you may have to return sooner, within days or weeks.

Repeated Tests

The baseline tests that you have at the initial visit are routinely repeated, in order to look for progression in your glaucoma.

When your eye doctor says that your eye pressure is under control, do you have to come back?

YES!

You still need to have regular follow-up appointments to manage your glaucoma. *The disease doesn't just go away, even if it is well treated.* This is true even if you have already had laser treatment or glaucoma surgery.

WHY?

Glaucoma is a chronic condition that does not go away. With treatment, glaucoma will either remain stable or get worse. Although there is no cure for glaucoma, we do have excellent treatment options that can help stabilize the disease.

Changes in Treatment

Glaucoma can get worse, even when the eye pressure stays well controlled. This could occur for a number of reasons. Sometimes, if the eye drops are not used as prescribed, eye pressure can rise and cause damage to the optic nerve. For example, some patients may only use drops the day before their exam. Their eye pressure may look good that day. When they don't use their drops regularly, however, their eye pressure will rise, and their optic nerve will be damaged. On the flip side, it could be that the treatment regimen *is* being followed, but the glaucoma has changed and become more aggressive.

In cases where eye pressure is not controlled, it could be that the eye drops that have been used for some time are not working as well anymore. In those who have had laser treatment for glaucoma, the results from some types of lasers are known to wear off over time. In cases where glaucoma is treated with surgery, early or late scarring can occur. This can cause the procedure to fail, with or without apparent symptoms. These scenarios are some of the reasons why glaucoma requires monitoring to check for any changes.

Take Action

Glaucoma is a chronic disease that does not go away, so you will continuously need to have follow-up care. If you miss an appointment, your doctor's office may call you to reschedule. If they don't, YOU have to take on the responsibility to call your doctor to reschedule that missed appointment. You want to make sure your disease is well controlled. You also need to make sure your eye drops and other medicines are in order. If you run out of any drop or medicine for glaucoma, it's imperative that you call your doctor for a refill or a new prescription. Glaucoma is an aggressive disease, and we need aggressive measures to fight it. This means we—doctors and patients—have to be informed and know what to expect, so we can manage it the best way we can.

TIP 8. KEEP YOUR MEDICAL RECORDS

As I wrote in Tip 7, "A picture is worth a thousand words." The same is true for any kind of information about your optic nerve if you have glaucoma. It is vital for you to be your own advocate. Make sure you have copies of your medical records and copies of pictures of your optic nerve, so you can share them as needed with your doctors.

A strong recommendation for you, especially if you travel from one place to another or change doctors, is to gain personal access to your medical records. You can do this by requesting your own personal copy. The state of your optic nerve when you are first diagnosed with glaucoma is the baseline for your eye doctors to follow over time. These tests (such as visual field tests or optic nerve fiber layer imaging) are in your medical record. It is more common nowadays to have access to electronic patient portals, where your exam report and tests are accessible. Paper copies, however, are also helpful. Especially try to keep the records from when you were initially diagnosed, so you and your health care providers can compare them over time with new results.

Important Information for Your Medical Records

Here is a list of information that I recommend keeping with your medical records:

- Baseline eye pressure at the time of diagnosis, before treatment began.

- Baseline evaluation of the optic nerve (cup-to-disc ratio notation and drawing).

- Any photographs of the optic nerve.

- First and last three visual field tests (if these aren't all available, then have the most recent ones on hand).

- Any nerve fiber layer imaging, such as OCT (see chapter 1).

- Any details on prior laser or surgical treatment for glaucoma.

In other words, it is imperative to get copies of both your old and updated medical records. Many medical practices do a good job of transferring your medical records. These records may not show up in a timely fashion, however. This commonly happens. If you have a set of your own personal records that you can supply on request, you will have less frustration if other medical records do not arrive on time, and you will have more control over your eye condition.

TIP 9. TALK TO YOUR FAMILY

Glaucoma Runs in Families

Glaucoma is a hereditary disease. This means that if you have glaucoma, so could someone you love. Anyone who is your blood relative has an increased risk of developing the disease as well. It is common for people to be diagnosed with glaucoma and not know of any family history associated with the disease. It is also possible, however, that you do have a relative with glaucoma who doesn't know yet that he or she has the disease, or does know it but did not relay that information to you for whatever reason.

Give the Gift of Sight

You can give the gift of sight to your family by letting them know you have the disease. This should be followed by strong encouragement for them to get their own eyes specifically checked for glaucoma. By sharing your diagnosis with your family members, you are allowing them to be proactive in preserving their vision. If you don't tell them, you're actually doing them a disservice, because the earlier they find out if they have glaucoma, the easier it is for them to treat it. If they have glaucoma, it is better to be diagnosed at an early stage, because early diagnosis with glaucoma is the key to proper management of the disease.

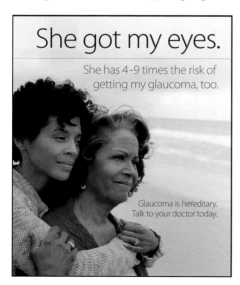

Figure 2.7. Family hereditary risk for glaucoma.

Glaucoma Family Facts

• A family history of the disease increases the risk of glaucoma 4 to 9 times, compared with those without glaucoma in their family.[13]

• Siblings are at the highest risk: approximately 10% of siblings of patients with glaucoma get glaucoma.[14]

• 1 in 8 relatives of people with glaucoma will also have the disease.[15]

So, at your next family gathering, make it a point to get everyone together and let them know about glaucoma (fig. 2.7). Stress how important it is for them to get their eyes checked to prevent vision loss in their life. You can also recommend that they read this book!

TIP 10. BE HONEST WITH YOURSELF

For Those Diagnosed with Glaucoma

If you are actively being treated for glaucoma, it is important to be honest with yourself. If you have been given a treatment regimen that includes using daily eye drops to help lower your eye pressure, it is of the utmost importance to keep up with that regimen. It is vital to put in your eye drops every day. The effect of the eye drops can wear off after so many hours, so forgetting your drops, or stretching out when you apply your drops, or not using your drops when going to certain meetings or events, can leave your eyes vulnerable to elevated eye pressure. You won't feel the eye pressure rise, but your optic nerve will feel it and slowly continue to deteriorate without your awareness. You don't want to lose your eyesight, and we, as your eye care providers, don't want that to happen to you, either.

Also, please understand that we do understand your situation. You, like many others, may have issues with your medication, such as:

"It costs too much."

"It makes my eyes irritated."

"It causes unpleasant side effects."

"It is difficult to remember to put it in."

All of these issues, and any others, are valid AND should be discussed with your doctor. Your doctor can change the regimen or address the issue, so that things will work best for you. It is much better to bring your concerns up for discussion than to be dishonest with yourself and your doctor and say that everything is fine. Remember, it's your vision that is at stake.

The good news is that there are typically other kinds of eye drops or other modes of therapy, such as light energy treatments with lasers and minimally invasive glaucoma therapies, that can be used to help control your glaucoma. Be real with yourself, and be open with your doctor. Let him or her know how you are really doing with the treatment regimen, so your doctor can come up with the best option for you.

For Those at Risk or a Glaucoma Suspect

You may have been told by a family member to get your eyes examined for glaucoma. Maybe you have already been examined before and told by a doctor that something in your eyes looks suspicious for glaucoma. This means you are a glaucoma suspect (not in the criminal sense— just in terms of your eye health!). Have you been hesitant to schedule that appointment for the evaluation? Maybe you see just fine and don't understand why you should bother to get checked out.

Well, maybe you *do* have glaucoma, also known as the "I see just fine, but I could go blind if I don't get screened" eye disease. Enough said.

Go get checked. Your sight is on the line.

TIP 11. KNOW THE RISKS ASSOCIATED WITH GLAUCOMA AND CATARACTS

Glaucoma is a disease that can develop at any age, but it is more common with increasing age. Another eye condition that also increases with age is cataracts (fig. 2.8). Although both conditions can lead to blindness,

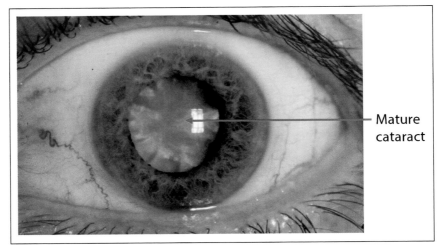

Figure 2.8. A mature cataract.

cataracts are curable, while glaucoma is not. A cataract is a condition in which the lens in your eye becomes cloudy. It is like looking through a fogged window. You cannot see well through a cloudy lens. Treatment for cataracts involves replacing the bad lens with a good one, a simple surgery. Glaucoma, on the other hand, results from damage to the optic nerve. Vision loss in glaucoma is irreversible. That is why it is crucial to screen for and treat glaucoma—to prevent further loss of vision.

Here's the Good News

Don't be discouraged when you hear that you have a visually significant cataract in addition to your glaucoma. In fact, there is good news for you! I have found that in some cases, the pressure-lowering effect can be greater when cataract surgery is combined with glaucoma surgery, compared with when glaucoma surgery alone is performed. This means that there may be a way to reduce or eliminate glaucoma drops if you are actively using them. There is a cutting-edge form of glaucoma surgery that has now been used for over a decade called minimally invasive glaucoma surgery, or MIGS. The types of surgical techniques used with MIGS allow a less invasive approach that is much faster and safer, compared with traditional glaucoma surgical techniques, yet still effective in lowering eye pressure. MIGS is easily coupled with cataract surgery, going through the same small incision to enter the eye. Also, the healing time for the combined surgery is very similar to that for just cataract surgery alone.

You're Not Alone

There are more than three million cataract surgeries performed every year, according to the Centers for Medicare and Medicaid Services. In about 20% of them, patients with cataracts also have glaucoma (known as co-morbid cataract and glaucoma) and are actively taking eye drops. If you have a visually significant cataract AND take drops for your glaucoma, you should ask your doctor about having combined MIGS and cataract surgeries (fig. 2.9). This presents a wonderful opportunity for many patients to conveniently have both procedures done at the same time. Seeing better, and also having better controlled glaucoma with fewer drops, equals a significantly enhanced quality of life!

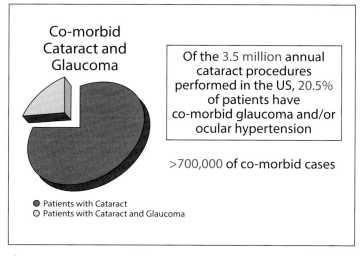

Figure 2.9. Cataract and glaucoma statistics.

TIP 12. MANAGE YOUR GLAUCOMA AND DRY EYES

Dry eye syndrome is a condition in which a person doesn't have enough useful tears to lubricate and nourish the eye (fig. 2.10). Dry eye is a common and often chronic problem, particularly in older adults. Common dry eye symptoms include:

- Burning eyes

- Irritated eyes

- Tired eyes

- Stinging eyes

- Gritty eyes

- Blurred vision

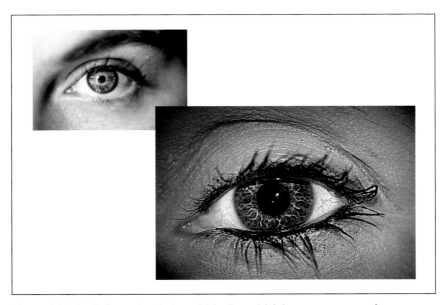

Figure 2.10. An inflamed or irritated "dry" eye (*right*), versus a normal eye (*upper left*).

- Red eyes

- Scratchy eyes

- Excess watering/tearing

Many factors can contribute to dry eyes, one of which is glaucoma drops. Many glaucoma drops have preservatives in them that can irritate the surface of the eye. This can create or exacerbate dry eye symptoms. Treatments for dry eyes aim to restore or maintain the normal amount of tears in the eye, both to minimize dryness and related discomfort and to maintain eye health. It is common for glaucoma patients to have mild redness in their eyes as a result of their glaucoma eye drops. Treating the eyes with the dry eye therapies described here can often reduce redness in the eyes.

Ways to Combat Dry Eyes in Glaucoma

Even though glaucoma drops are used to prevent vision loss, you don't have to have dry, red, uncomfortable eyes. There are many options to treat these dry eye symptoms. Some of the options can include the following:

1. *Switch the types of medication you use.* There are different classes of glaucoma medications and, typically, several different brands within each class. It is not always clear which kind of drop will be best tolerated by each individual patient. Some eye drops can be combined into one bottle. Talk to your doctor to find the best tolerated and most effective medication for you.

2. *Try preservative-free drops.* Another option is to switch to a preservative-free form of glaucoma drops. There are several drops now on the market that are preservative-free and still can lower eye pressure and reduce symptoms of dry eye.

3. *Use glaucoma laser treatments.* Using light energy, through a laser procedure, is also an option. There are several laser procedure options, typically performed in an office setting, depending on your type of glaucoma. This form of treatment, in turn, has the potential to reduce or eliminate the need for glaucoma drops and reduce dry eye symptoms. A recent study called the LiGHT Trial showed that a laser treatment called SLT was effective in reaching the target eye pressure in 95% of nearly 400 patients for 3 years. None of them required glaucoma surgery to lower eye pressure, compared with 11 patients who required surgery in the group receiving only eye drop therapy.[16] From this evidence, there has been a shift to considering glaucoma laser treatments as the first therapy to try.

4. *Ask about minimally invasive glaucoma surgery (MIGS).* With the advent of MIGS, options for glaucoma surgery are now offered earlier. This can be helpful, especially when glaucoma is at an early or moderate stage, eye drops are not tolerated, and laser treatment has not been fully effective. The use of MIGS avoids the potential risks involved with traditional glaucoma surgeries, such as a trabeculectomy or a tube shunt (see chapter 1). MIGS can effectively decrease eye pressure, and many patients can reduce or fully stop their need for glaucoma drops after a successful MIGS procedure.

If the best option, according to your doctor, is to stay on your current glaucoma regimen, dry eye symptoms can still be treated in a number of ways.

- *Over-the-counter artificial tears.* This is typically the first-line treatment for dry eyes. Preservative-free artificial tear solutions are recommended, because they don't have additives that could further irritate the eyes.

- *Prescription dry eye medications.* There are several classes of eye medications that can be used to help create more tear production, improve the quality of the oils within your eyelids, or reduce inflammation that can sometimes be the cause of the dry eye symptoms.

• *Punctal plugs.* To keep your natural tears in your eyes longer, silicone or dissolvable gel-like plugs can be placed in your tear ducts, where the tears normally drain. This creates a blockade, so more natural tears wet your eye, helping reduce dry eye symptoms. Imagine that the tears in your eye are like water in a leaky bottle. To maintain the same amount of water in the bottle, you can either pour more water in the bottle (use artificial tears) or plug the hole (use a punctal plug).

• *Vitamin supplements.* Omega-3 fatty acids are known to help improve the quality of the oils within the eyelid glands. This, in turn, can play a role in reducing tear film evaporation.

• *Warm compresses.* A washcloth moistened with hot water or a microwave-heated eye mask can provide heat to help soften oils, open oil glands within the eyelids, and aid in reducing dry eye symptoms.

• *Lid scrubs.* These cleaners can help decrease inflammation and remove bacteria and debris from around the surfaces of the eyes.

• *LipiFlow or iLux.* These are in-office procedures that use a thermal pulsation system to open and clear blocked oil glands. The procedure allows the body to resume the natural production of oils needed for tear film.

• *BlephEx.* This is another in-office procedure. It involves using a handpiece with a gentle exfoliator tip to remove debris and film on the eyelid margin, which can clog natural oil glands and prevent the release of oils that coat the surface of the eye. This procedure can decrease symptoms of dry eyes, such as itchy, scratchy eyelids and eye redness.

As you can see, there are many options for dry eye treatments. You can learn more about some of these dry eye treatment strategies on my iGlaucoma Patient channel on YouTube, at https://bit.ly/3B3iVzJ. Ask your doctor which treatment you should start with to help your eyes feel better. Remember, just because you have glaucoma doesn't mean you should have dry, red, angry eyes.

Dry Eye Self-Care Treatments to Start Now

You can take the following steps, starting right now, to reduce symptoms of dry eyes:

1. *Blink:* Remember to blink regularly when watching television, reading, or staring at a computer screen for long periods of time. Lack of blinking will dry out the surface of the eye.

2. *Follow the 20/20/20 rule:* Every 20 minutes, look at least 20 feet away for 20 seconds. This will help you avoid eyestrain and fatigue.

3. *Add moisture:* Increase the humidity in the air at work and at home. Using a desktop humidifier or a room humidifier can help provide moisture.

4. *Use eyewear:* Wear sunglasses outdoors, particularly those with wraparound frames, to reduce exposure to drying winds and the sun. This can also be helpful in the car when air or heat is blowing toward your face.

5. *Drink water:* Stay hydrated by drinking plenty of water (8 to 10 glasses) each day.

3

Keeping It Real
Real Patients, Real Advice

Having glaucoma can feel very lonely at times because others around you may have trouble understanding life as seen through your eyes, and it can be difficult to explain. Part of the journey of living your best life with glaucoma should include sharing experiences with others who also have glaucoma. When you open up and reach out to others with this disease, you will realize that, in fact, you are not alone, and that there are many out there like you going through similar experiences. This realization can put you at ease, give you encouragement, and even allow you to learn something that can greatly benefit you and others.

Understanding this concept, and also knowing that some of you reading this book may not yet have had the opportunity to reach out to someone, I did it for you! I have asked some of my actual patients, who I know are battling with glaucoma but living vibrantly, to share their stories. They have various stages of glaucoma: from mild, to moderate, to severe. I have enjoyed having the privilege to take care of them, and they have each inspired me with their glaucoma journey, life challenges, and triumphs. I thought it would be a great addition to this book of advice from a glaucoma doctor's perspective to include real stories and real advice from actual glaucoma patients. I hope the next few pages will have a significant positive impact on helping you live the best life, despite having glaucoma.

For Charmaign Vauters, glaucoma was a gradual process through which she found herself with a loss of vision.

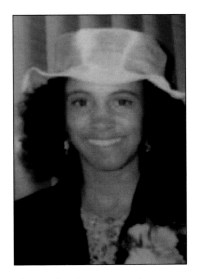

Charmaign Vauters, a glaucoma patient of Dr. Constance Okeke.

■ Looking back at before my glaucoma diagnosis, I had only Saturday nights to sit and watch Pandora on the big TV in the sitting room. I started noticing that the vision in one eye was not as keen as the other, and I was doing more of listening to the show than watching, but even then I would try to rationalize it with diet and exercises.

The glaucoma diagnosis was given to me clearly and in all seriousness, but I found it hard to place myself that day.

My glaucoma diagnosis made me realize how valuable my eyes were to me; they were my superpower. Early on as an organ donor, it was the organ I specifically chose to donate one day. But now it felt like spring was behind me, and I was entering autumn.

And so I took the diagnosis seriously, and even though I had never had to take medications daily, I took up the responsibility of taking up to 5 doses of eye drops per day to prepare for successful eye surgery.

Looking back, I should have gotten prescription glasses immediately after the diagnosis; I felt the glasses added protection to my eyes. I even made a proactive decision during the pandemic to wear eye protection indoors in public spaces, and when I was asked why I wore a mask and a shield, I would say, "My mask protects you, your mask protects me, and my shield protects me."

Through this stage in my life, I have learned three essential things about glaucoma: if it is not diagnosed or treated, it will result in blindness; secondly, the effect of glaucoma, which is loss of sight, is irreversible; and with proper diagnosis and treatment, eyesight can be saved before damage is done.

My doctor, Constance Okeke, MD, is the best support resource. The literary and visual resources she produces at her office, Virginia Eye Consultants, are the best; I always refer to them in my pursuit to stay educated and informed.

My best advice to anyone recently diagnosed with glaucoma is that you educate yourself, no information is a waste, and seek out the best professional medical treatment while taking extreme care to protect your sight and eyes.

Establish an eye care regimen with a professional health expert experienced in the field and stay committed to your eye care. When I moved to a new city, I thought about establishing care in my county, but I realized that I was already enjoying the best medical care. These types of important decisions will help you care for your eyes better. Basic decisions like wearing sunglasses also help; before my diagnosis, I never wore sunglasses, but now I always have them on me, wearing them outdoors or indoors in public places. During the pandemic, I always had my shield up.

Regarding medications, I started to lose count of how many times I had taken my eye drops, so I got creative and playful about staying on schedule, always thinking about the adverse effects of not taking my medications.

My sight is my hidden treasure in plain sight, and I once set my sights on taking "recreational" helicopter lessons after I retired. The main attraction to this was the knowledge that this required specially trained pilots. I was told that to operate a helicopter, each extremity has a distinctly assigned task different from others—that is, each arm and leg had to perform tasks wholly distinguished from others. It was fascinating to me; I thought, as a senior, what a wonderful way to keep the brain sharp. But the harsh reality is if you are losing your sight, whether you know it or not, there will be a day when you will be exempt from doing what you love or aspire to do because your sight is going or gone.

For my family, I told them about my diagnosis, and subsequently, they took the initiative to schedule eye examinations; and I am proud to say as a result, they can all quote their eye pressures. With constant care, there has been an improvement in mine, too. ▪

Arlene Kessell didn't notice any changes in her vision before and after she was diagnosed with glaucoma.

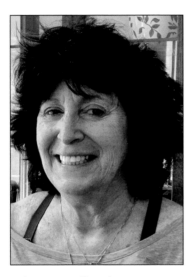

Arlene Kessell, a glaucoma patient of Dr. Constance Okeke.

▪ When my ophthalmologist informed me of her diagnosis, I was taken aback, shocked, stunned. The diagnosis had to be a mistake, but it wasn't. My initial [elevated] eye pressure was in the mid-twenties, and that was a serious cause for alarm. I would never have suspected I suffered from glaucoma, as I thought it occurred only in the elderly . . . I was in my early forties. I noticed absolutely no change in vision. After the diagnosis, my situation was thoroughly explained to me, and I was overwhelmed, honestly frightened for the worst-case scenario: loss of sight. I recall asking, "What do we do now? What's your plan?" My alarm was so intense, I felt we had to hurry to make this vision thief disappear immediately, but there is a catch, you see. This thief is a permanent guest who stays for the rest of my life. I was anxious to begin treatment, to learn as much as possible about this cursed disease (aren't all diseases cursed?), and follow my doctor's advice perfectly.

My glaucoma has been my uninvited visitor for about twenty-five years. If you imagine a pie, cut across it to create an upper and lower half. My upper halves of this pie form my blind spot. I can see, I can read, but I am somewhat aware I am missing half the picture. As a result of this vision loss, I frequently and painfully hit my head and forehead. When playing with my dogs in my tree-filled yard, I am forever hitting tree limbs, branches, bird feeders hanging from branches. I hit my head often on/in my car when loading the rear of the front seat area. I also see nothing on the left side of my world. I have learned to adapt as well as possible.

I have been a perfect glaucoma patient; I cannot afford not to be if I want to maintain my vision, as much vision as possible.

If you are recently diagnosed with glaucoma, be concerned, very concerned. The loss of vision is not noticeable to you; you are losing peripheral vision and are not even aware of the loss. Use your drops! Apply them correctly! Follow your doctor's direction religiously!

I look forward to Dr. Okeke's appointments because of the very nature of glaucoma; I may not be aware of a change in my eye pressure or a loss in my visual field, but my doctor can detect this during the appointment. The best resource I have found is my ophthalmologist. Ask questions!

My advice to family or caretakers of glaucoma sufferers is simple: make sure drops are applied correctly—that is, at correct times of day, in the correct eyes (occasionally, a drop is applied to one eye only); keep all ophthalmology appoint[ment]s! Make sure all eye drop refills are current!

The top three things the glaucoma patient must keep in mind are (a) glaucoma can cause you to go blind; (b) a spike in your eye pressure can still occur when you are flawlessly applying your eye drops; you will feel helpless, [but] (c) be thankful for every day you can see. Trust your doctor implicitly.

To someone who has recently been diagnosed with glaucoma, I would say to listen to your ophthalmologist, be attentive, do not be hesitant to ask questions. Follow a regimen for your eye drops. Never skip a dose! Again, trust your doctor implicitly.

As regards to families, make sure all family members have a glaucoma test annually. This is not to be taken lightly. Keep in mind that you might believe you have no vision problems; however, that is the very nature of this thief of sight! Glaucoma does run in families! But the good news is it can be controlled and suppressed not to disrupt activities throughout one's life.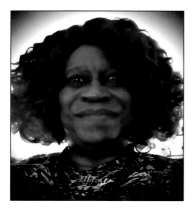

Rosalind Quaye didn't notice any signs that would have suggested she had glaucoma.

There were absolutely no signs such as pain, eye swelling, itching, or seeing double. I only became aware of its silent theft after my nearsighted mother told me of her referral visit to an ophthalmologist and diagnosed glaucoma. My mother reported the specialist inadequately informed her of the disease but did discuss its hereditary aspect and advised her [about] alerting family members. She notified me several years later, at which time I wore corrective eyewear due to pathological myopia.

Rosalind Quaye, a glaucoma patient of Dr. Constance Okeke.

As in any stage of myopia, I could not see the distant fate of glaucoma-specific depreciated vision, which I probably had then; no signs exhibited until later receiving specialist findings, revealing advanced stage glaucoma. Glaucoma is a thief and a robber! I felt violated and victimized, violated by a hereditary vision stealer, victimized by its effectiveness and personal burden of complicity attributed to inappropriate eye care decision-making.

I did not see it coming, and glaucoma, having no respect for vision's state, stole beyond suffering higher-degreed myopia (worse than 20/400 uncorrected vision). When detected in its advanced stage, glaucoma had upgraded injury to my already damaged optic nerve by partnering with other thieves and robbers, perpetrators such as life-threatening diabetes, hypertension, and inflammation.

The diagnosis of the disease was clearly articulated, but a comprehensive synopsis of the disease was omitted. At first, I did not take the diagnosis of glaucoma seriously due to a chronic addiction to distrusting physicians. A personal inability to detect any vision change beyond my 45-year comfortability with nearsightedness, crowned with years of ignoring annual eye examinations, contributed to prideful behaviors.

Just seeing was enough for me. Quality of sight did not enter my exceedingly large portfolio of "priority" things to do. A new pair of glasses was a treat. I saw how to, without assistance: read the Holy Bible and secular books; perform acts of maternal and neighborly love; travel to and from gainful employment; navigate sidewalks and cross busy streets; watch out for human predators and other creeping things; identify and run from danger; see and hail a cab; travel by ferry, bus, train; satisfy legal and medical secretarial job duties.

During those years of ignorance, I thrived considerably as a young, family-oriented, purpose-driven, vivacious, "indestructible" super single mom! Able to defeat any Goliath, glaucoma was NOT a prioritized concern; in fact, I just did not have time for a daily regimen of a time-consuming 10 minutes for administering eye medications and keeping scheduled follow-up appointments, with wait times exceeding three hours.

I did not take the diagnosis of glaucoma seriously at all; I settled for the grandeur vision correction afforded—enjoying a false sense of confidence. Oblivious to an unseen vision future and an impending drastically altered quality of life, I remained in the dark, proudly declaring to others, "An ounce of prevention is better than a pound of care!"

An attitudinal change has led to full compliance with keeping all scheduled and emergent eye appointments and, respectively, diligent obedience to specialists' advice. Personal experience with glaucoma, staying informed on groundbreaking news, and applying readily available tips on the disease motivate information-sharing on personal health and eye cares.

My advice on living well with glaucoma to someone recently diagnosed is to schedule taking your eye drops on a timely basis daily; alert your care team of allergic reactions to any medication; ask family members and friends to assist with transportation, cooking, and household chores; develop healthy eating and a regular physical exercise regimen; maintain good rapport with your glaucoma management team, keeping all appointments and following their care instructions.

If you are family to someone who's been diagnosed with glaucoma, be sober minded. Do not take your vision or the vision of others, including family members and neighbors, for granted. Love them as you love yourself and show this by communicating your experience with glaucoma and how it can impact their sight, and taking immediate bold, proactive steps toward obtaining professional consultation.

Additionally, I counsel all family members and neighbors to educate themselves on glaucoma to develop sensitivities necessary for understanding behaviors or challenges of afflicted persons. Take advantage of the portfolio of businesses, resources, and apps supporting the blind and vision impaired.

Through my situation, I have learned glaucoma is an eye disease that results from varying degrees of damage to the optic nerve, which leads to permanent loss of vision. Vision loss is gradual, painless, prolonged, and unbeknownst to the patient—necessitating keeping regular and annual eye care appointments for early specialist detection and management intervention. Glaucoma, inherited or acquired, makes everyone at risk for developing the disease; however, persons having a family history of glaucoma are more susceptible.

If you've recently been diagnosed with the disease, I suggest that you have faith in God! He can heal you, and His grace is sufficient to show you His perfecting strength in your weakness. Give conscientious attention to measures of prevention, maintenance, and optimizing good health and eye care. This same consideration must be given when one's sight becomes compromised by the presence of any eye disorder and disease.

Glaucoma runs in families, so I emphasize that you do not delay in seeking a professional ophthalmology consult. Be consistently and fully compliant with specialist management instructions. Stay abreast of current glaucoma-specific news and related medical issues. Proactively share your awareness and experience with others. Thank God for the ability to do all of the above. ▪

Roger Vann Smith was also interviewed about his experience with glaucoma.

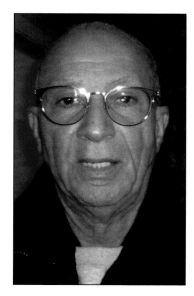

Roger Vann Smith, a glaucoma patient of Dr. Constance Okeke.

▪ There was no sign whatsoever that would have led me to believe I had any eye disease, including glaucoma. . . . At the time of my diagnosis, I did not know such a disease existed. The purpose of my initial professional medical services visit to my then-ophthalmologist was to have an eye examination and receive transition lenses.

The first thoughts I had were "Glaucoma," and "How it would bear upon my professional service two-year contract one way or another?" The diagnosis was given to me clearly, since my elder sister is and was a practicing medical doctor in New York City, my legal domicile; I knew to ask questions regarding any gray area I required further comprehension on.

I took the diagnosis and prognosis seriously. Why? My doctor informed me that if the glaucoma was not successfully treated and controlled, I would lose my eyesight. Furthermore, Dr. Kolsky informed me he could not professionally advise me to be in Saudi [Arabia] unless my glaucoma was medically controlled. Otherwise, I could lose vision in at least one eye. Ergo, my ailment potentially had an economic bearing on both my immediate family and me. Therefore, my employer was immediately contacted, and my movement was placed on hold for several months.

Glaucoma is said to be hereditary; I can't change my genes to avoid this disease. So I just follow the treatment procedures. So, my advice to people diagnosed with glaucoma is to secure professional providers with complete confidence in their professional services. Also, pressure your federal legislators for more research and development with curing this disease, and insurance coverage universally throughout this our nation for everyone under an extended ongoing amendment of the Affordable Care Act applied to all states, like Social Security.

Caring and concerned medical doctors such as Constance Okeke and Martin P. Kolsky have been the best resources and support I've had. My advice to families or caretakers of people with glaucoma is not to take the matter lightly. While you have sight, protect it by following the professionally advised procedures. If payment for services or medications is a problem, confidentially speak with a servicing physician for assistance. Things can be done, possibly including taxation write-offs if necessary and hardship medications from pharmaceutical entities doing well financially [that] can afford some write-offs.

My diagnosis and the treatment of glaucoma have taught me to take my medications as prescribed, keep to appointments, inform my physician of situation changes, and avoid depression through prayerful faith, family, and love.

If you've recently been diagnosed with glaucoma, know that it's a brave new world. You can get over it by being positive. If you believe it is a lemon, then make lemonade out of it. Otherwise, think of it as an apple pie. Take a slice and enjoy the ride while doing everything you are supposed to do medically. Where you can't, then I suggest, as I have, to consider asking for help with prayer.

Glaucoma runs in families, so should you be amid a family which holds periodic reunion gatherings, recommend to the reunion planning committee to invite, if possible, an ophthalmologist.

Many sufferers of glaucoma can live comfortably with it as long as they control it and follow treatment procedures. One essential element is having faith as opposed to fear.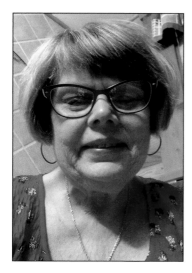

June Hart talked about her experiences with glaucoma being added to other eyesight issues.

In retrospect, I probably had some symptoms. I was already struggling because of my detached retina surgery for that eye; I remember having problems with light, and my eyes were red. When I came for my follow-up session, I met Dr. Okeke; it was said that the pressure in my eye was too high.

The diagnosis given to me was clear. I remember going to the mailbox one day in the sunlight, and the light was killing my eyes; they were so itchy and red that I had to get them checked out. I took the diagnosis seriously because of what I had already been through with my retina and permanently losing my sight in one eye, and all the struggles with surgery. I did everything I was told to do willingly, because I don't know what I would do without my sight. . . . I know I'd survive; I've learned to do so many things by feeling since I don't have any eyesight in my left eye, but glaucoma affected my peripheral vision, and I struggled with that.

June Hart, a glaucoma patient of Dr. Constance Okeke.

My advice to any person diagnosed with glaucoma is that you need to research it and know more about it. Be aware of the damage so that it doesn't get to the point where it's irreparable. Take it seriously, listen to your doctor, and take the medication as directed. If you go blind due to damage to the optic nerve, you can't get your sight back.

Early on, I knew something was going on with my eyes, and I was a little scared. You don't want to be diagnosed with something terrible, but then you have to learn to accept things and just do what you need to do for your illness and then move forward. That's what I've done. Generally, men have it worse; they never go to the doctor, their wife has to make the appointment, make him go. People say they don't have time to go to the doctor. Yeah, but you don't have time to lose your sight, either.

Talking to people helped me a lot. If you've ever struggled without sight or glaucoma or anything with your retina or whatever, you know you don't hesitate to go to the doctor; you need to go. I would suggest that if somebody was just diagnosed with it, they get involved in a support group or other patients who have gone through this and get advice from them and testimonies from them. That way, it would help them on their journey, because it makes you aware that you're not alone.

I tell my family always to have their eyes checked. Glaucoma is passed genetically. You might not know you have it, so make sure you go to the doctor to get checked, especially if someone in your family has been diagnosed with it. I have nearsightedness in my family, and I remember struggling as a child trying to see, and then my grandmother took me to the eye doctor to get glasses. Then I'd feel some changes in my eyesight, and I'd think, "It's just because I'm nearsighted."

I have learned that the damage that glaucoma does to your optic nerve is irreparable and that you need to take it seriously, do your drops as needed, go to the doctor, and have checkups as required. If you're having struggles to make sure you tell your doctor everything going on, it might not seem like it's something big, but it could be. You also have to be aware and be responsible for your health, and go to your doctor.

If you've been recently diagnosed with glaucoma, my advice is that you take it seriously and try to stay positive. I have had many trials through this process, from very scary times, but I lean on God and know that He gives me the strength. He continues to help me push forward each day to a new tomorrow with hope and praise.

People don't want to ask questions sometimes, because they think they're stupid questions, but when it comes to your health and your eyesight or anything like that, no question is stupid, because if you don't ask that question, you're not going to find out an answer.

Conclusion

I hope you have found much value in the words you have read in this book. This book is designed for multiple audiences: diagnosed glaucoma patients, patients without glaucoma but who are at risk, eye care providers who take care of these patients, and the caregivers, family, and friends who take care of loved ones with glaucoma. I wish I had the time to talk to each of you individually and share these messages. Nonetheless, I hope that my thoughts have been made clear.

Just to recap, here are some take-home messages about glaucoma:

1. Don't ignore the signs of glaucoma.

2. Do the simple "Cover Your Eyes So You Can See" test for a quick screening of an eye problem.

3. If you are diagnosed with glaucoma, accept the disease.

4. Conquer your fears. Don't despair. Have hope. Technology is advancing, and you can take action to preserve your vision.

5. Take glaucoma seriously. It doesn't go away because you ignore it.

6. Ask your doctor questions. Be prepared for each exam.

7. Know what is expected.

8. Keep your medical records. Take control of your health.

9. Talk to your family members. Glaucoma runs in families.

10. Be honest with yourself, and be open with your doctor.

11. Know the risks associated with glaucoma and cataracts. There are great technologies that can help if you have both glaucoma and cataracts.

12. Manage your glaucoma and your dry eyes. Just because you have glaucoma doesn't mean that your eyes have to stay uncomfortable. There are options to help.

If you have found value in this book, please share it with others, as the message of glaucoma awareness needs to be spread far and wide—locally, regionally, nationally, and globally. If, by writing these words, I can help even one person preserve their vision and prevent them from going blind, then it was well worth the effort, and I will be eternally satisfied. Knowledge is power. Use it, and we'll preserve global vision together.

Acknowledgments

First and foremost, I am grateful to my husband, Richard Okeke, who not only helped in editing this book but was also integral in every step—from the book's inception to the reality of production. I am grateful to my children, Izu, Ify, and Obi, who are a constant source of inspiration and encouragement.

I would like to thank those who contributed to the reviewing, editing, and beta reading of my work and helped put together the final touches for the book. Thank you.

To Vanessa Caceres, Stefan Edemobi, June Hart, Shanon Joynes, Arlene Kessell, Audrey Lazar, Rosalind Quaye, Roger and Faye Smith, Charmaign Vauters, and Harold Wheeler—your comments and suggestions were extremely helpful.

I am appreciative of the Virginia Eye Consultants' doctors, staff, and patients. My experiences with you inspired and supported the work within the book.

I am endlessly grateful to God. Through Him, all things are possible.

Resources

Guide to Putting in Eye Drops Correctly

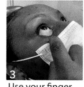

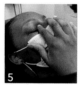

1. Wash your hands first.

2. Tilt your head back and look up at the ceiling.

3. Use your finger to pull down your lower eyelid to create a pocket.

4. Gently squeeze one drop from the bottle into the pocket.

5. Gently close your eyes and press on the inside corners of your eye.

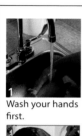

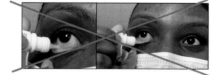

6. Blot away excess drop on skin.

Do NOT touch the tip of the bottle to your eye, your fingers, or anything else.

How to instill eye drops.

Caregiver's Guide

When a loved one is diagnosed with glaucoma, it can be stressful. If you are caring for someone who has glaucoma, you may wonder how you can make that person's life easier, particularly if they have lost or are losing sight. We hope this guide helps dispel some of the myths surrounding glaucoma and leaves you feeling prepared to help your loved one on the glaucoma treatment journey. Here are a few facts you should know about glaucoma and how some real-life glaucoma patients describe it. The photos in this section are representative of glaucoma patients.

Glaucoma is a disease that damages the eye's optic nerve:

- It usually happens when fluid builds up in the front part of the eye.

- The extra fluid increases the pressure in the eye, damaging the optic nerve.

Glaucoma is sneaky:

- Primary open-angle glaucoma, the most common type of glaucoma, is usually painless, has no symptoms, and causes no vision changes at first.

- Nearly half of Americans with glaucoma do not even know that they have it.[17]

- People with glaucoma sometimes believe they have good vision, because they can see things in the center of their visual field but are not aware of things in their peripheral vision.

Here is how some real-life glaucoma patients describe it.[18]

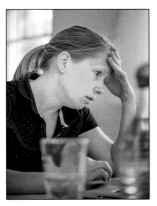

"I was still seeing well enough, but one evening I was out walking when a man suddenly appeared in front of me. It was, as they call it, a classic 'jack-in-the-box' moment: one minute my way was clear, and the next minute he popped suddenly into the middle of my field of view."

"[The doctor] had me stand across the room from her and asked me to focus one eye on her nose and tell her how much of her body I could see. I couldn't believe what I saw. She only existed above the shoulders and below the hips. Her torso wasn't there. I literally felt sick. It was the first time the reality sunk in."

THE EMOTIONAL IMPACT OF GLAUCOMA

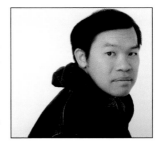

Patients with glaucoma often go through a wide range of emotions. Knowing what your loved one might be feeling can help you be patient and understanding. Here are some fears, similar to what I have heard from my patients.

Fear of going blind

"There is no light at the end of the tunnel. You don't know what is going to happen to you. Maybe you will go blind tomorrow, and the whole world is dark."[19]

Feelings of hopelessness
"I was going to do art, but there's no point at all."[20]

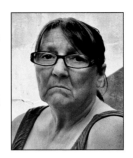

Frustration with vision changes
"Reading the paper . . . I would just give up and say, 'You know, it's not worth it.' "[20]

Desire to talk with others with glaucoma
"Some of them have a long period of time managing this disorder, so they can tell me how to deal with it."[19]

Loss of independence
"I think it's emasculating—you know, for a man to lose his driver's license."[20]

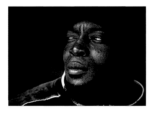

Worry for their friends and families
"What worries me is my only son. I hope the tragedy [of having glaucoma] won't happen again."[19]
  "I really hate asking people for lifts."[20]

Social difficulties
"I'm not very good at identifying people's faces. That's gotten worse over the years . . . my wife has to explain, 'That's so-and-so's wife.' "[20]

Withdrawal
"I've sort of stepped down from positions of responsibility, really, being on committees and that sort of thing, because I just felt I was really unreliable and I knew I was going to have to go in for more surgery or something. That really rocked me."[20]

   People with glaucoma can experience anxiety or depressive symptoms. The ways in which you help your loved one with glaucoma manage these symptoms is what's important.[21]

What You Can Do

Here are some tips to help you in your caregiving:

- Reassure your loved one that glaucoma is treatable.

- Patients with glaucoma can still do many of the activities they have always enjoyed if they are willing to follow their eye treatment plan and visit their specialist regularly.

- Make sure your loved one goes to his/her follow-up visits.

- Offer to drive your loved one and take notes during doctor appointments.

- Help your loved one stick to his/her medications and treatment plan.

- Your loved one may feel overwhelmed by new medication regimens and instructions, so offer to help with the treatment plan.

- Ask for help.

- Enlist other family members and friends to rotate responsibilities and build a strong network of support.

- Talk about the emotional effects of glaucoma.[22]

- Receiving a diagnosis of glaucoma can cause anyone to experience a range of negative emotions, from grief and shock to anger and depression, so it is important to talk about your and your loved one's emotions and feelings. By treating it as a family issue, you can help your loved one feel supported.

- If your loved one with glaucoma is a family member, schedule a complete eye examination for yourself.[23]

- The most common type of glaucoma, primary open-angle glaucoma, is hereditary. If a member of your immediate family has glaucoma, you are at a much higher risk than the rest of the population.

The good news is that with early detection, and by diligently following a treatment plan, most people with glaucoma will not lose their sight.[24]

Additional Resources for Glaucoma Caregivers

Bright Focus Foundation
https://www.brightfocus.org
The Bright Focus Foundation offers a "Disease Toolkit" for glaucoma, including pointers and how-tos, such as "Tips to Manage Caregiver Stress."

Rides in Sight
https://www.ridesinsight.org
Rides in Sight provides a database of transportation programs that can assist in getting your loved one to his/her follow-up visits.

Homemods.org
https://www.homemods.org/resources/
Homemods.org offers information on how to modify homes to make them safer for people at risk from falls and other injuries.

Health in Aging
https://www.healthinaging.org
Health in Aging furnishes caregiving how-tos and an e-newsletter for a broad range of conditions, including glaucoma.

Guide to Finding a Glaucoma Specialist

Here are a few tips to keep in mind if you are in the process of choosing a specialist to diagnose or treat glaucoma. Following these tips can help you find a competent, caring doctor.

1. *Find someone experienced in treating glaucoma.*
There are a variety of websites that list glaucoma providers, which can help you narrow down who is located in your area and who might be right for you or a loved one.

The American Glaucoma Society (AGS) is composed of glaucoma specialists dedicated to sharing clinical and scientific information for the benefit of patients, colleagues, fellows, and residents. As a member, I often use the AGS website as a reference tool for my patients who are relocating to other areas to find new doctors. You can find a glaucoma specialist by doing the following:

- Go to the AGS website, at americanglaucomasociety.net.

- Click on the link at the top of the page that says "Find a Doctor."

- Enter the relevant zip code and search your desired geographic radius.

Learn more about additional resources for finding doctors on the Glaucoma Research Foundation's website at https://www.glaucoma.org/treatment/finding-a-doctor.php.

Although there are several types of doctors who specialize in eye care—including opticians, optometrists (OD), and ophthalmologists (MD/DO)—ophthalmologists are trained medical doctors who have the most expertise in glaucoma. The training for an ophthalmologist includes 4 years of college (receiving a bachelor's degree), 4 years of medical school (receiving an MD or DO degree), a 1-year internship, and 3 years of ophthalmology residency training, where they obtain thousands of hours of medical and surgical training. Some ophthalmologists go on to further specialize in glaucoma care through a yearlong fellowship training. The members of AGS have all received glaucoma fellowship training.

The training for an optometrist includes 2–4 years of college (a bachelor's degree is not required) and 4 years of optometric school (receiving an OD degree). Some optometrists go on to obtain a year of medical training working alongside an ophthalmologist, though this is not required. When glaucoma is mild or controlled with medications, optometrists can be a good resource to manage glaucoma, and they commonly work with glaucoma specialists to monitor glaucoma patients and help with post-operative management. Optometrists will refer glaucoma patients to ophthalmologists when there are medical issues that are moderate to severe, are difficult to control, or are in need of more advanced treatment, such as laser treatment or glaucoma surgery.

2. *Come to your first visit prepared with questions.*
By asking questions, you make your health care (or care for a loved one) a top priority. Having questions also has another purpose: you get a better sense of the doctor's empathy and knowledge. Because glaucoma is a chronic disease, you most likely will see this doctor many times. You want to choose someone with whom you feel comfortable asking questions.

3. *Reflect on your first appointment.*

After you have an initial appointment with a provider, think back on your experience or talk about it with someone you trust. Were you comfortable in the office? Were the staff and the doctor friendly? What was the wait time like? Could you see yourself going there long term? Answers to these questions can help reveal if that office is a good match for you. If it's not, don't be shy about finding another provider.

Additional Resources for Glaucoma Patients

Although living with vision loss isn't easy, there are many resources and apps available to help with daily tasks and let you better understand what glaucoma is. Here is a list of some of those resources and apps.

ONLINE GLAUCOMA RESOURCES

Note: Several of the resources below also have information in Spanish.

American Academy of Ophthalmology's Eye Health
https://www.aao.org/eye-health/
https://www.aao.org/eye-health/diseases/what-is-glaucoma/
The American Academy of Ophthalmology is the largest association of ophthalmologists in the world, with more than 30,000 members. It has an EyeSmart website. The first URL focuses on consumer information about eye health. The second URL is about glaucoma.

American Glaucoma Society
https://www.americanglaucomasociety.net/patients/
The American Glaucoma Society is a group geared toward glaucoma providers, but its website also has an educational section for patients.

American Optometric Association

https://bit.ly/3nNmKnO/

The American Optometric Association's website has a vision rehabilitation fact sheet, "Finding Help for Vision Impairment, Low Vision, and Blindness."

Glaucoma Research Foundation

https://www.glaucoma.org

https://www.glaucoma.org/news/podcasts/audio-podcasts.php

The Glaucoma Research Foundation specializes in information about glaucoma care. The second URL features its patient-geared podcast, which includes episodes such as "Lifestyle Choices and Glaucoma" and "Stem Cell Treatment for Glaucoma."

Hadley

https://hadley.edu

The mission of Hadley is to create personalized learning opportunities that empower adults with vision loss or blindness to thrive—at home, at work, and in their communities.

Prevent Blindness

https://www.preventblindness.org

https://www.preventblindness.org/glaucoma/

Prevent Blindness focuses on better eye care and eye health. Information on the second URL focuses on glaucoma.

National Eye Institute

https://www.nei.nih.gov

https://www.nei.nih.gov/learn-about-eye-health/eye-conditions
-and-diseases/glaucoma/

The National Eye Institute is part of the federal government's National Institutes of Health and is heavily involved with eye research and clinical trials. Find its glaucoma information at the second URL.

iGlaucoma Patient YouTube Channel

https://bit.ly/3B3iVzJ

The iGlaucoma Patient YouTube Channel is a resource of free educational videos and helpful guides about glaucoma and issues that pertain to glaucoma patients. This channel was created by Dr. Constance Okeke to further the spread of knowledge about glaucoma for patients and their loved ones.

Helpful Glaucoma Apps

Check to see if the apps below are available for your smartphone. In addition to these specific apps, there also are a variety of magnifying glass apps for both Apple and Google Play. Some of these also provide additional light when using the app.

AARP Caregiving

This is a free app that empowers caregivers with information on how to effectively care for a loved one, coordinate care with other family members and friends, and keep track of appointments and medications.

Be My Eyes

This innovative app connects people who are blind or have low vision with sighted volunteers who can help them with daily tasks. For instance, you may want to know what color a shirt is, if your milk has expired, or what button to use on a remote control. Help on the app is available in 185 languages.

EyeDropAlarm

This app allows you to set an alarm to remind you to take your eye drops. The names of certain glaucoma drops are embedded in the app, so you can easily select the names that apply to the drops you use.

EyeNote
Designed by the US Bureau of Engraving and Printing, EyeNote can "read" US currency and let you know its denomination.

Glaucoma Notebook
This app lets patients set phone-based alarms to remind them to use their drops. You can also use the app to keep track of your intraocular pressure.

Medisafe
This free smartphone app tracks your prescriptions and reminds you when it's time for a refill.

Pocket Glasses Pro
This is a magnifying app to help you see things more closely without glasses. There are other apps for both Apple and Google Play with similar functions.

Seeing AI
Use this app to recognize and narrate text that is detected by your smartphone camera. This app also can read bar codes, name the colors of articles of clothing, and perform other tasks that can help those with vision issues.

Spotlight Text
This app helps those with low vision read e-books. The app has several books on its site that are ready to read.

References

1. Benowitz L, Yin Y. Optic nerve regeneration. Arch Ophthalmol. 2010;128:1059-1064.

2. Javitt JC, McBean AM, Nicholson GA, Babish JD, Warren JL, Krakauer H. Undertreatment of glaucoma among Black Americans. N Eng J Med. 1991;325:1418-1422.

3. Muñoz B, West SK, Rubin GS, Schein OD, Quigley HA, Bressler SB, Bandeen-Roche K. Causes of blindness in a population of older Americans: The Salisbury Eye Evaluation Study. Arch Ophthalmol. 2000;118:819-825.

4. Pekmezci M, Bo V, Lim AK, Hirabayashi DR, Tanaka GH, Weinreb RN, et al. Characteristics of glaucoma in Japanese Americans. Arch Ophthalmol. 2009;127:167-171.

5. Varma R, Chung J, Foong AWP, Torres M, Choudhury F, Azen SP, et al. Four-year incidence and progression of visual impairment in Latinos: The Los Angeles Latino Eye Study. Am J Ophthalmol. 2010;149:713-727.

6. Quigley HA, West SK, Rodriguez J, Munoz B, Klein R, Snyder R. The prevalence of glaucoma in a population-based study of Hispanic subjects: Proyecto VER. Arch Ophthalmol. 2001;119:1819-1826.

7. Chen S-J, Lu P, Zhang W-F, Lu J-H. High myopia as a risk factor in primary open angle glaucoma. Int J Ophthalmol. 2012;5:750-753.

8. Mastropasqua L, Lobefalo L, Mancini A, et al. Prevalence of myopia in open angle glaucoma. Eur J Ophthalmol. 1992;2:33-35.

9. Tielsch JM, Sommer A, Katz J, Royall RM, Quigley HA, Javitt J. Racial variations in the prevalence of primary open-angle glaucoma: The Baltimore Eye Survey. JAMA. 1991;266:369-374.

10. Tham Y-C, Li X, Wong, TY, et al. Global prevalence of glaucoma and projections of glaucoma burden through 2040: A systematic review and meta-analysis. Ophthalmology 2014;121(11):2081-2090.

11. Quigley HA, Vitale S. Models of open-angle glaucoma prevalence and incidence in the United States. Invest Ophthalmol Vis Sci. 1997;38;83-91.

12. Wittenborn JS, Zhang X, Feagan CW, Crouse WL, Shrestha S, Kemper AR, et al. The economic burden of vision loss and eye disorders among the United States population younger than 40 years. Ophthalmology. 2013;120:1728-1735.

13. Vajaranant TS, Wu S, Torres M, et al. The changing face of primary open-angle glaucoma in the United States: Demographic and geographic changes from 2011-2050. Am J Ophthalmol. 2012;154:303-314.e3.

14. Wolfs RC, Klaver CC, Ramrattan RS, van Duijn CM, Hofman A, de Jong PT. Genetic risk of primary open-angle glaucoma: Population-based familial aggregation study. Arch Ophthalmol. 1998;116:1640-1645.

15. Wolfs RGC, Klaver CCW, Ramrattan RS, Van Duijn CM, Hofman A, de Jong PTVM. Genetic risk of primary open-angle glaucoma. Arch Ophthalmol. 1998;116:1640-1645.

16. Gazzard, G. Konstantakopoulou E, Garway-Heath D, Garg A, Vickerstaff V, Hunter, R, et al. Selective laser trabeculoplasty versus eye drops for first-line treatment of ocular hypertension and glaucoma (LiGHT): A multicentre randomised controlled trial. The Lancet. 2019;393:1505-1516.

17. Carduner S. Patient's guide to living with glaucoma. VisionAware. https://visionaware.org/your-eye-condition/glaucoma/patients-guide-to-living-with-glaucoma/. Accessed August 10, 2020.

18. Lovett J. Joe Lovett: Activist and documentary filmmaker. https://visionaware.org/emotional-support/personal-stories/eye-conditions-personal-stories/joe-lovett/. Accessed August 10, 2020.

19. Pei-Xia Wu, Wen-Yi Guo, Hai-Ou Xia, Hui-Juan Lu, Shu-Xin Xi. Patients' experience of living with glaucoma: A phenomenological study. J Adv Nurs. 2011; 67: 800.

20. Glen FC, Crabb DP. Living with glaucoma: A qualitative study of functional implications and patients' coping behaviours. BMC Ophthalmol. 2015:128.

21. Johnston D. Dealing with the emotional angst of vision loss. BrightFocus Foundation. https://www.brightfocus.org/macular-glaucoma/chat/dealing-emotional-impact-vision-loss/. Accessed August 10, 2020.

22. BrightFocus Foundation. Caring for someone else. BrightFocus Foundation. https://www.brightfocus.org/macular/caregiving/. Accessed August 10, 2020.

23. Glaucoma Research Foundation. Are you at risk for glaucoma? Glaucoma Research Foundation. https://www.glaucoma.org/glaucoma/are-you-at-risk-for-glaucoma.php. Accessed August 10, 2020.

24. The Glaucoma Foundation. Treating glaucoma. The Glaucoma Foundation. https://glaucomafoundation.org/aboutglaucoma/treating-glaucoma/. Accessed August 10, 2020.

Philanthropy

Thank you for buying this book. Congratulations! By purchasing this book, you have joined the fight against glaucoma blindness. Your efforts are helping two great organizations that are working toward a glaucoma cure and active surgical treatment for those with financial hardships.

I am donating some of the proceeds of my book royalties to the following organizations:

The Glaucoma Research Foundation

The American Glaucoma Society (AGS) Cares Program

The Glaucoma Research Foundation (GRF) is a nonprofit organization that is dedicated to improving the lives of glaucoma patients and funding innovative research to find a cure. I am proud to be a long-standing GRF Ambassador and provider of educational materials from the GRF to my glaucoma patients. For additional details about glaucoma diagnosis and treatment and to learn more about GRF's research efforts, please visit their website at www.glaucoma.org and request or download their free, newly revised booklet, "Understanding and Living with Glaucoma."

The AGS Cares Program is a public service program dedicated to delivering surgical glaucoma care at no cost to uninsured or underserved patients who qualify for such care. The glaucoma care is provided by members of a national network of volunteers: glaucoma surgeons who are active or provisional AGS members. I am proud to be a long-standing AGS member and volunteer for the AGS Cares Program. To learn more about the AGS Cares Program, go to https://www.americanglaucomasociety.net/patients /ags-cares/.

Index

Page numbers followed by *f* and *t* are references to figures and tables, respectively.

IMAGE CREDITS

CHAPTER 1. All figures are courtesy of Dr. Constance Okeke, with the following exceptions. **page 4:** Courtesy of KeithJJ (pixabay.com), https://www.needpix.com /photo/655164/soccer-football-soccer-players-kick-kicking-soccer-ball-game-competition -action/; **pages 6–9:** Courtesy of Mangdesain; **page 10, *bottom right*:** Courtesy of Willis Lam, https://commons.wikimedia.org/wiki/File:Golden_Donut_Cinnamon_Sugar _Doughnut_(30801404415).jpg; **page 14, *top left*:** Courtesy of Clker.com, http://www .clker.com/clipart-23701.html; **page 14, *top right*:** Courtesy of Kissclipart.com, https: //www.kissclipart.com/weak-national-government-clipart-united-states-of-eiufp9/; **pages 18–22, *images on the right only*:** Courtesy of Pixabay.com, https://pixabay.com/photos/ energy-saving-lamp-1340220/; **pages 24–25:** Courtesy of Mangdesain; **page 29, *top*:** Courtesy of Needpix.com, https://www.needpix.com; **page 29, *bottom*:** Courtesy of Piqsels .com, https://www.piqsels.com/en/public-domain-photo-sxeuz/; **page 30:** Courtesy of Pixabay.com, https://pixabay.com/photos/eye-check-optometry-doctor-optician-5091177/; **page 31:** Courtesy of Bright Focus, https://www.brightfocus.org/glaucoma/article/how-eye -pressure-measured/; **page 33, *top*:** Courtesy of FotothekBot, https://commons.wikimedia .org/wiki/File:Fotothek_df_n-10_0000776.jpg; **page 38:** Courtesy of Mangdesain.

CHAPTER 2. page 50: Courtesy of Pxfuel.com, https://www.pxfuel.com/en/free-photo -eeecc/; **page 52:** Courtesy of Nohat.cc, https://nohat.cc/f/photo-of-man-covering-his -face/4577996564332544-201812131338.html; **page 54:** Courtesy of Pixabay, https: //pixabay.com/photos/hospice-hand-in-hand-caring-care-1793998/; **page 56:** Courtesy of Maxpixel.net, https://www.maxpixel.net/Give-Candle-Open-Prayer-Hands-Candlelight -Pray-1926414/; **page 57:** Courtesy of Maxpixel.net, https://www.maxpixel.net /Man-Mood-Face-Eye-Emotion-People-Message-Look-164218/; **page 60:** Courtesy of Maxpixel.net, https://www.maxpixel.net/Psychiatrist-Discussion-Doctor-Consultation -Patient-5710152/; **pages 65, 68–69:** Courtesy of Dr. Constance Okeke; **page 70:** Courtesy of the Centers for Disease Control and Prevention, https://www.cdc.gov /conjunctivitis/about/symptoms.html.

CHAPTER 3. All photographs are courtesy of the subjects.

CAREGIVER'S GUIDE. page 97, *top*: Courtesy of Needpix.com, www.needpix.com //photo/802511/adult-annoyed-blur-burnout-concentration-facial-expression-frustrated -girl-indoors/; **page 97, *bottom*:** Courtesy of Sheldon Botler Photography/Aclew, https: //commons.wikimedia.org/wiki/File:AlbertLew_Sophisticate.jpg; **page 98, *top*:** Courtesy of Needpix.com, www.needpix.com/photo/433574/sad-woman-expression-stress-depressed -unhappy-grief-caucasian-head/; **page 98, *bottom*:** Courtesy of Needpix.com, www .needpix.com/photo/438791/people-black-homeless-black-people-person-african-young -adult-american/.

ABOUT THE AUTHOR

Dr. Constance Okeke is a board-certified ophthalmologist who is committed to educating her patients and the community about how to fight glaucoma blindness.

She received her undergraduate and medical degrees from Yale University and trained in ophthalmology at the Wilmer Eye Institute of Johns Hopkins University. She completed her glaucoma fellowship training as a coveted Heed Research Fellow at the Bascom Palmer Eye Institute of the University of Miami, and then went on to earn a Master's of Science in Clinical Epidemiology at the University of Pennsylvania.

Dr. Okeke has practiced ophthalmology, with a specialty in glaucoma and cataract surgery, for more than 20 years. She has received numerous awards and honors, including the prestigious recognition of being voted by her peers to *The Ophthalmologist*'s global top 100 female Power List for 2021 and global top 100 combined male and female Power List for 2022. Currently, she is an assistant professor of ophthalmology at Eastern Virginia Medical School and the lead glaucoma specialist at CVP—Virginia Eye Consultants in Norfolk, Virginia. In addition to teaching, she sits on the editorial advisory board of the journals *Glaucoma Today*, *CollaborativeEYE*, and *Glaucoma Physician*. Dr. Okeke also has two educational YouTube channels that feature glaucoma surgical techniques: iGlaucoma, which is geared towards eye care professionals, and iGlaucomaPatient, which is aimed at patient education and support.

As part of her efforts to educate doctors in emerging techniques in the area of minimally invasive glaucoma surgery (MIGS), she wrote her first book, *The Building Blocks of Trabectome Surgery: Patient Selection*. Dr. Okeke is a leading expert, pioneer, and trainer in the area of MIGS on national and international levels.

Dr. Okeke makes her home in Hampton Roads, Virginia, with her loving husband and three children.

For more information about Dr. Okeke and her work, visit her website at www.DrConstanceOkeke.com.

HEALTH & WELLNESS BOOKS FROM HOPKINS PRESS

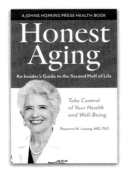

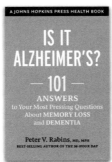

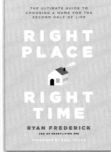

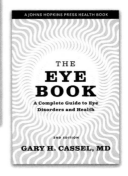

Honest Aging

An Insider's Guide to the Second Half of Life

Rosanne M. Leipzig, MD, PhD

"[This] new handbook on aging is full of clear, practical advice that will make the second half of your life safer, more productive, and more enjoyable. It is essential reading for anyone who is growing older or whose loved ones are growing older—in other words, for all of us!"—Martha Stewart

Is It Alzheimer's?

101 Answers to Your Most Pressing Questions about Memory Loss and Dementia

Peter V. Rabins, MD, MPH, best-selling author of The 36-Hour Day

A medical expert answers your common questions about memory loss, causes of\ dementia, diagnosis, prevention, treatment, and more.

Right Place, Right Time

The Ultimate Guide to Choosing a Home for the Second Half of Life

Ryan Frederick, CEO of SmartLiving 360; Foreword by Paul Irving

Wondering where to live in your later years? This strategic and thoughtful guide is aimed at anyone looking to determine the best place to call home during the second half of life.

The Eye Book

A Complete Guide to Eye Disorders and Health, 2nd ed.

Gary H. Cassel, MD

The Owner's Manual for Your Eyes: The most comprehensive guide to taking care of vision.

Available in Large Print

press.jhu.edu

 @JHUPress

 @HopkinsPress

 @JohnsHopkinsUniversityPress

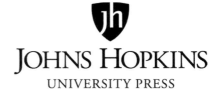